WORKING FOR
A HEALTHIER
AMERICA

WORKING FOR A HEALTHIER AMERICA

edited by:

Walter J. McNerney
Blue Cross/Blue Shield
Associations

BALLINGER PUBLISHING COMPANY
Cambridge, Massachusetts
A Subsidiary of Harper & Row, Publishers, Inc.

International Standard Book Number: 0-88410-718-3

Library of Congress Catalog Card Number: 80-20143

Printed in the United States of America

Library of Congress Cataloging in Publication Data

Blue Cross Association.
  Working for a healthier America.

  Papers presented at the Blue Cross/Blue Shield Associations 50th
Anniversary symposium, in Washington, D.C., 1979.
  Includes index.
  1. Medical care — United States — Congresses.   2.   Public
health — United States — Congresses.   3.   Medical policy —
United States — Congresses.   I.   McNerney, Walter J.   II.   Blue
Shield Associations   III.   Title.
RA395.A3B545 1980   362.1'0973   80-20143
ISBN 0-88410-718-3

CONTENTS

LIST OF FIGURES

LIST OF TABLES

ACKNOWLEDGMENTS

The greater part of the credit for the store of intelligence and wisdom readers may find in these pages should go to the distinguished members of the jury that selected recipients of our Blue Cross and Blue Shield fiftieth Anniversary National Health Achievement Awards. The jurors, who are all authors of comments included in this volume, were John A. D. Cooper, M.D., president of the Association of American Medical Colleges; David A. Hamburg, M.D., president of the Institute of Medicine, National Academy of Sciences; Julius B. Richmond, M.D., assistant secretary of the U.S. Department of Health and Human Services and surgeon general, U.S. Public Health Service; and Nathan J. Stark, undersecretary, U.S. Department of Health and Human Services. Their contribution brought us the award recipients who are named elsewhere here and whose essays are the hard bones and long muscles of this book, along with addresses by Ambassador Brewster, Secretary Harris, and White House Assistant Stuart Eizenstat. Also assisting with the design of the Anniversary Symposium and the preparation of this publication were Duane R. Carlson, vice president, communications, of the Blue Cross and Blue Shield Associations, and Robert M. Cunningham, Jr., a consultant to the associations.

INTRODUCTION

WORKING FOR A HEALTHIER AMERICA

Walter J.McNerney
President, Blue Cross and
Blue Shield Associations

Fifty years ago, the concept of prepayment of the costs of medical care was born when Justin Ford Kimball, administrator of Baylor University Hospital in Dallas, organized the first group hospitalization plan for Dallas school teachers. The persuasive economic logic of prepayment was quickly picked up and adapted to the needs of other communities, at first specifically for hospital care and soon for physicians' services as well. Throughout the half-century of growth of this Blue Cross and Blue Shield concept, which has given rise to a nationwide network of Plans protecting more than 100 million American men, women, and children and paying $45 billion a year for the hospital and medical services they need, the principles established in those early years have prevailed—nonprofit organization, community service, public as well as provider representation in the governance of local Plans, and service benefits.

As the theme for the fiftieth anniversary observance, the Blue Cross and Blue Shield Associations and the Plans chose to emphasize what has been, and will remain, the guiding direction of the prepayment concept: "Working for a Healthier America," the rubric under which this volume has been prepared. It is no coincidence that the essays and comments here,

3

focused as they are on several fields of public policy—financing and delivery of health services, public health, and education and research related to the health of Americans—are all as concerned with problems as they are with accomplishments. It is not just chance that they all deal in one way or another with what are seen as likely developments for the future, or that they are not only lacking in any notable reverence for what some of us view as the considerable contributions of the Blue Cross and Blue Shield Plans over the years but in some instances are inclined to find fault. The contributors were invited to examine the state of the art in their several disciplines without reservation and to envision what were likely to be the developments affecting the health of future generations of Americans.

The authors of the principal essays were chosen by a painstaking process. Aware that the health status of the population is determined not only by the reach and quality of medical and hospital care but, equally important, by the quality and nature of the environment, the community, and the education and welfare systems, an anniversary committee representing the Blue Cross and Blue Shield Associations and the Plans decided that there should be a series of National Health Achievement Awards for noteworthy contributions in health care delivery and research, health economics, preventive medicine and public health, occupational and environmental health, and medical and health education. The basis of the awards would be the impact of the candidates' achievements on the health of the population, both now and as projected for the future. These were the terms described to a jury of outstanding leaders in medicine and health affairs, who reviewed the accomplishments of several hundred nominees and made the final selections. Recipients of the awards, and the achievements for which they were recognized, were:

The Honorable Wilbur J. Cohen, for his inspired leadership of the movement resulting in legislation making health care services available and affordable to the elderly and the poor;
Eli Ginzberg, Ph.D., for his lasting contributions to the knowledge of the economics of health care, health manpower, and planning, and health care financing;

James A. Shannon, M.D., Ph.D., for his masterly and productive administration of the complex scientific research activities of the National Institutes of Health;

Donald A. Henderson, M.D., for his management of the World Health Organization's worldwide smallpox eradication program, resulting in virtual elimination of that deadly disease;

H. Jack Geiger, M.D., for his development of a new concept of community health care based on concern for the needs of populations for food, income, housing, and welfare services, as well as health care;

Norton Nelson, Ph.D., for founding the Institute of Environmental Medicine at New York University and guiding its development as the leading center for scientific studies of the impact of environmental agents on health; and

Walsh McDermott, M.D., for his memorable contributions as a teacher of physicians and as editor of a textbook dealing with the entire panorama of the knowledge of disease.

The award recipients were asked to prepare the papers that are the principal contents of this volume. In condensed form, these papers were presented at a Blue Cross and Blue Shield Associations fiftieth Anniversary Symposium, held in Washington, D.C., in December 1979 as the concluding event of the anniversary year. Also presented there were comments by distinguished authors, which have been selected by the editor and included here, and addresses by U.S. Ambassador to the United Kingdom Kingman Brewster, Jr., U.S. Secretary of Health and Human Services Patricia R. Harris, and Stuart E. Eizenstat, special assistant to the President for domestic affairs.

As I examined the thoughtful explorations of needs, problems, and possible future directions in the several professional fields represented here, I was reminded of a statement in an essay written a generation ago by the French theologian and philosopher Teilhard de Chardin: "Like nervous passengers in a ship or an aircraft who turn their eyes away from the ever-moving emptiness of sea or air, we generally shun the prospect of the future into which we are launched. Clinging to the more solid framework of what has already been acquired, and of the past, we try to forget the bewildering domain of possibilities in which we are swallowed up." Our authors here can scarcely be regarded in this light. On the contrary, it seems to me they have looked realistically at the bewildering domain, sorting out the possibilities and the problems with a confidence rooted in the successes they have achieved in the past and are still achieving. Necessarily, achievers are more concerned with what is than with what may be, more with what can be managed than with what can be imagined, and more with the near term than with anything more remote.

Peering out at the realm of future possibilities, some of the communications technologists have been telling us that the new microminiaturized computers, in combination with new imaging technology providing two-way, coast-to-coast linkages, should make it possible within a short time for telemedical consultations, for example, to be conducted by specialists in New York or Boston, say, for patients in New Mexico or Alaska, practically on demand. Hospital rounds and professional seminars could enlighten the practitioner in Montana along with the residents at the bedside with the Harvard professor. Laboratory, radiological, cardiological, and other medical data could be processed for the whole country in a handful of centers, and the same kind of technology could permit many, if not most, of the diagnostic and therapeutic procedures now conducted in our hospitals to be performed in patients' homes.

Will any of this actually be done? Probably some of it will be, but I suggest that these and other applications will lag behind technological capabilities and reach boundaries of acceptability that the futurists don't always foresee, constrained by countervailing forces that are firmly embedded in our culture. Thus the health services' planning experience of the past fifty years, from the original report of the Committee on the Cost of Medical Care in 1932 to the Health Systems Agencies of the 1970s, should have taught us that local pride and local autonomy give way slowly, if at all, to regionally centralized services, however persuasive the economic logic. The slow growth over an even longer period of the formulation that was called "contract practice" a generation ago and is now known as Health Maintenance Organization (HMO) should have taught us that the person-to-person value system of medical care, which has been in place since the time of Hippocrates, is not easily displaced. Like the technology, these things, too, will change, though probably not as rapidly or extensively as some of the oracles have been suggesting.

Here and elsewhere, we have learned about the growing interest of industry in the health of the work force, awakened in part by the ever-increasing knowledge of the occupational and environmental hazards to health, and in part, certainly, by the constantly mounting cost of paying for the care of sick or injured employees—something those of us in the Blue Cross and Blue Shield organization are acutely aware of. So industry— and this is true of labor as well as management—is seeking and establishing programs aimed at keeping employees well and teaching them how to keep themselves well, and programs aimed at holding down the costs of getting them well when they get sick or hurt. Interest in all these programs has been increasing rapidly in the past year or two, and forecasters tell us that in time the large corporations will buy into, or buy out, the medical care system, the way the auto industry bought out the parts industry a generation ago.

Now, I suppose it is possible to read the future that way, for some corporations are contracting with professional standards review organizations to monitor care of employees in hospitals and encouraging the formation of HMOs in areas of major concentration of employee populations. But as to how far these goals are likely to be pursued, we must look again at the cultural restraints and at the difference between the medical care system and the auto parts industry. Medical care might be purchased or paid for by industry in the aggregate for employees and their dependents, but medical care is provided for patients by physicians one at a time, and the collective values are as different from the distributive values as the computer is from the stethoscope. Volume, efficiency, and cost weigh heavily on one side, and quality, precision, and care are ascendant on the other. The key to an appropriate balance of these values during the next decade—and possibly for the long term as well—must be found in some combination of public regulation and an infusion of market forces and incentives into the health care system. Both are present to some extent and have been evolving slowly over time; the task will be to speed up the process without either sacrificing quality to achieve efficiency or using quality as a screen to hide inefficiency.

Our disenchantment with government regulation—to state the proposition as delicately as possible—has evoked the conviction that answers must lie in the free play of market forces among providers of health care services. I would agree that we do need more incentives, more options, and more competition of the right kind, but we must never lose sight of the difference between the collective and distributive values.

In this search for the desired balance of values, there are essential roles for government, providers of services, industry, labor, health insurers, and consumers. What are needed in all of these sectors are people who are not only experienced and competent but also imaginative enough and brave enough to test new methods of organizing, financing, and delivering services—with innovative programs, fresh forms, and improved relationships of the components. Fifty years ago there were plenty of critics around to tell the pioneers of the prepayment concept for health services that their ideas weren't needed and wouldn't work, and there are critics on all sides now to tell us that we don't need anything new. But we can honor our Blue Cross and Blue Shield predecessors most by being willing to do what they did: Take the risks required to try other ways of doing things.

One encouraging sign for the future is that recently there has been so much new public awareness of the importance of good health habits—not just in the jogging phenomenon and what has been called the "fitness mania," but also in notable changes in food consumption, smoking and drinking habits, and exercise programs. Especially significant are the many activities initiated and underwritten by industry to identify employees who are considered to be poor health risks and to offer constructive intervention and education programs aimed at health improvement. These are good starts. Together with our concerns about national health insurance, cost, planning, and technology, they raise new public questions about priorities in our use of resources. For example, how shall we strike a proper balance between curative and preventive medicine? What should be the goals, and the content, and the level, of health education of the public? Whose job should it be? How much can be spent, and with what results? On these and other pertinent questions there is conflict within the professional community, with many of our most revered authorities in the biological sciences questioning whether the evidence justifies any major investment in health education of the public, for example, and insisting that under any circumstances there should be no diversion of resources from biomedical research. And no matter how these issues may be resolved over the years (and the answers will not come readily), these are not "either/or" questions. We are seeking a middle ground—not a reversal of values but an added value, not less medicine but more prevention. Here is a critical role for doctors and hospitals, but with support from industry, labor, government, insurers, schools, and community groups.

An essential element in all of this is voluntary enterprise. It has been local, voluntary initiative and energy and resources that have fueled the development of the health services in America, and it is only this vitally influential "third sector" that can resolve the issues confronting us now and for the future. Our pursuit of expansion and specialization in the 1950s and 1960s permitted issues of access and financing to arise, and the legislation that resulted has had a dampening effect on the spirit of voluntarism. Under the pressures of cost and regulation, the private sector has become defensive. We have no reason to be so: The initiatives, the innovations, and the progress have come from voluntarism, not from government. The voluntary system, not government, pioneered in introducing third-party payment, prospective reimbursement of providers of services, areawide planning, HMOs, ambulatory surgery, and home care. It was voluntary institutions that created medical audits, utilization review, shared services, and multi-institutional management systems. It was private insurers, not public programs, who first linked finance to planning, utilization controls, and medical necessity, and who have turned the spotlight of public attention onto the wellness movement.

Whenever these and other voluntary innovations have developed too slowly, they have needed some of the public prodding that is now being applied. But they were voluntary initiatives nevertheless. There has always been a place for government resources and governmental authority and standards, and there will be such a place in the future—establishing goals and limits and helping to finance services wherever voluntary resources may fail to reach. What is needed is an effective partnership of public and private interests, capitalizing on what each sector can do best. Forging such a partnership while preserving the estate of voluntarism that is our heritage is our most important task for the future, as we work for a healthier America.

PUBLIC POLICY: FINANCING AND DELIVERY OF HEALTH SERVICES

1 SERVICES, HEALTH SERVICES, AND THE GENERAL WELFARE

Eli Ginzberg, Ph.D.
Professor of Economics, Graduate School of
Business, Columbia University

Eli Ginzberg, Ph.D., is the A. Barton Hepburn Professor of Economics at the Columbia University Graduate School of Business. Through his books, articles, lectures, consultations, and public appearances, he has made many contributions to the advancement of knowledge in the economics of health care, health manpower, health planning, and health financing. The author of numerous books, including A Pattern for Hospital Care, Men, Money and Medicine, *and* The University Medical Center *and the Metropolis, Ginzberg has been an effective critic of both the public and private health care delivery systems, offering many proposals for change. He has served on many commissions and committees and as a consultant to government. A medical consultant to the Hoover Commission, Ginzberg served as an advisor to the Commission on Chronic Illness, as chairman of the National Commission for Manpower Policy, as director of the New York State Hospital Study, on the Science Advisory Board of the U.S. Air Force, and as chairman of the Commission on Studies of the 1960 White House Conference on Children and Youth.*

To look ahead to the end of the century and suggest ways whereby the U.S. medical care system can continue to make significant new contributions to the well-being of the American people is tantalizing: too long for simple extrapolations of present trends and not long enough to enable the prognosticator to disregard the structures in place. Consider playing the reel backward—to the last years of President Eisenhower's term of office—with Kerr-Mills just having been placed on the statutes; the battle over Medicare not yet joined; Medicaid not even a gleam in the eye of Wilbur Cohen; the AMA uptight about a lot of things, but still dominant; the biomedical community riding high; the term "cost containment" not yet coined; and considerations of health manpower of concern only to a few specialists. Within the last twenty years the most powerful nation on the face of the globe was tripped up by the Viet Cong guerrillas, Arab sheikhs, an Iranian mystic, Cuban soldiers on the African continent, PLO terrorists, and still others who, in an earlier day, would not have commanded the attention of the most junior departmental official, much less the secretary of state, the joint chiefs of staff, or the President.

With the health care sector accounting in 1979 for about 10 percent of national income, with a current expenditure level of $200 billion and 7 percent of total employment with approximately 6.4 million workers, there is little need to apologize for applying the term "industry" to health care activities and for considering what economics might contribute to improving our understanding of the allocation of resources and the delineation of public policy.

Perhaps no apology is needed in making use of economics to assess health care, but caution is definitely called for. Economics is a way of thinking, nothing less and nothing more. It is just twenty years since Selma Mushkin opened the first conference of health economists at the University of Michigan. In my presentation there, I warned that health economics was more than curves and computers and that it consists of one part economic theory and nineteen parts institutional knowledge and political judgment. I still believe this is the correct ratio.

The ratio holds not only for the mixed economies of the West but also for the centrally planned economies of the Soviet bloc. Within the recent past, my research group at Columbia University, the Conservation of Human Resources Project, received a group of Russian economists who, when they inadvertently learned that we were involved in research in medical economics, wanted to discuss nothing else. They reported that they had not found a way to improve the productivity of their health care system; they saw no end to the absorptive capacity of the health sector to devour scarce resources, particularly manpower; and they pressed us to tell them of any successes that the United States might have had in reducing the flow of resources into its health care system.

The United States and the Soviet Union are clearly not alone in their concerns about the efficacy and efficiency of their health care systems. High orders of uncertainty, questioning, and criticism are part and parcel of the experience of all developed countries, from Sweden to Australia, as well as of countries in the middle-income range, from the Philippines to Nigeria.

The basic assumption underlying this analysis stipulates that the political leadership, and its economic advisers, have an inadequate understanding of the dynamics of the production and distribution of services, a shortcoming that leads them to errors in evaluating what is, and in designing policies of what might be. Accordingly, I will deal sequentially with three interrelated themes: how one should think about services; the implications of such conceptual clarifications for assessing health care services; and the further consequences of such clarifications for setting health care goals for the end of the century and beyond, and the directions of reform required to achieve them.

Great contributors to human thought such as Adam Smith, whose *Wealth of Nations* was acclaimed by the eminent nineteenth-century essayist Thomas Buckle as the most important book in the history of mankind—the Bible alone excepted—make their impact by exploring a hitherto unrecognized or underemphasized idea. The market (Smith), class conflicts (Marx), and the unconscious (Freud) represent such contributions. But the shapers of the mind usually introduce error even while they are adding an important element of truth. So it happened that Adam Smith defined as "unproductive" all effort that did not result in a material output. The piano maker is productive; Horowitz when he plays to an audience of several thousand is not. This is not the place to explore why Smith made this sharp distinction between productive goods and unproductive services, beyond noting that in his effort to explicate "the nature and causes of the wealth of nations" he saw expenditures on services as failing to add to the capital stock. But whatever his rationale for the distinction, economic theory and conventional thought have been misled and confused—a confusion that is still with us.

The labor employed in the production of a house, an automobile, or a refrigerator, according to Smith, is productive since it results in a material output. But the crew of a ship carrying holiday seekers to the Caribbean, the surgeon who performs a lifesaving operation, and the telephone repairman are not. Their efforts do not result directly in material output. Although economists more than a hundred years ago recognized the limitations of this Smithian dichotomy and sought to escape from it by focusing on the "utility" (satisfaction) that people derive from spending their money on either goods or services, the old distinction lives on. The head of one of the largest U.S. manufacturing corporations is concerned that only one out of four of his quarter-of-a-million-person work force is engaged directly in the production of goods. The other three work on planning, design, engineering, advertising, marketing, financing, transportation, and still other "overhead functions" that the chief executive office views as "nonproductive"!

A second dichotomy, this one between investment and consumption, also rooted in Adam Smith's seminal work, contributes further to intellectual confusion. In Smith's view, increasing the wealth of nations depends on saving some part of current output and investing it to expand the factors of production, which alone can lead to larger output in the future. But Smith observed that consumption is the goal of economic activity. The reconciliation that economists have attempted goes as follows: One should reduce consumption today in order to enjoy a higher level of consumption tomorrow. Fine, but as the writer of Ecclesiastes recognized, the pursuit of ever higher levels of consumption makes little sense in a world in which the days of man are limited and the more they have, the more they want. Nowhere is the dilemma between investment and consumption more patent than when leaders seek to justify a higher level of expenditures on education, on the ground that those who graduate from college or professional school will enjoy higher lifetime earnings, or when critics of the steeply rising outlays for medical care emphasize that a disproportionate amount is spent on individuals who are no longer productive members of the labor force. These observations have a point, but they surely do not provide adequate criteria for determining the scale of educational and medical services in an affluent democracy.

The comparisons between productive and unproductive labor and between investment and consumption are clues, but nothing more, of the difficulties that policymakers and economists face in dealing with services. For the last hundred years and more, their dominant model has been a manufacturing enterprise geared to the production of physical output. We lack the conceptual apparatus to think sensibly about services, particularly professional services, a critical component of which are those for health care. One way to move ahead is to explore schematically how services differ from goods with respect to selected dimensions such as production, distribution, consumption, investment, employment, and social control. Such clarification is a precondition for assessing the potentialities and limitations of reshaping the health care sector so that it can become more responsive to the needs of the American people.

The essence of a successful manufacturing enterprise is an aggregation of physical capital and a work force that can be specialized to a point where increasing output can be achieved at declining unit costs. A critical component is the undertaker, the entrepreneur, who is skillful in combining the two, operatives and labor-saving machinery. The classic manufacturing unit uses a large number of semiskilled workers easily replaceable from the large pool of potential workers looking for a job. Over time, the employer seeks to substitute additional machinery for labor with the aim of cutting his costs.

At this point it is essential to make two distinctions that have not been part of conventional analysis until recent years—the distinction between consumer and producer services and the further distinction between services and professional services. As the terms "consumer" and "producer" suggest, there are services that meet the demands of consumers—such as waiters, workers in dry-cleaning establishments, and bus drivers. In contrast, there are "producer" services that are critical inputs for assisting employers in producing output—such as management consultants, corporate lawyers, investment bankers, and accountants.

For the most part, the skill level of those engaged in the production of consumer services tends to be lower than that of those who play an intermediate role by contributing to output while it is still under the control of the manufacturer or, more correctly stated, is not being bought by the final consumer. But this distinction as to relative skill levels must not be pressed too hard. The firm that has a contract to maintain machines for a large manufacturer may use a considerable number of technicians, and some providers of consumer services, such as lawyers and physicians, are often among the most highly educated and trained. The term "professional services" is utilized in the present situation to emphasize that well-trained professionals—physicians—are at the apex of the health care system, although they are assisted by many of lesser education and training.

The output of professional services follows a different tack from the output of material goods. Here the human resources input is critical—the professional who has specialized in a particular arena, such as the architect who designs commercial buildings in suburban areas or the lawyer whose practice is primarily directed to antitrust litigation. Although capital inputs may facilitate the work of professionals—architects use advanced systems of reproducing drawings and antitrust lawyers may have recourse to a computer to identify relevant cases in preparing their briefs—ideas, rather than physical capital, dominate their work.

There is a further distinction between the production of goods and professional services: In the former case, successive units of output are more or less identical. The machines control the transformational process. But the design for a group of office buildings or the briefs for successive antitrust suits are never cut from the same mold. The distinctive elements predominate.

Where distribution is concerned, the differences between goods and professional services are even greater. Goods can be produced for inventory and can be shipped, usually substantial distances, unless they are of great bulk and relatively low value, such as brick. Professional services involve interaction between producer and consumer. A physician must examine a patient in order to treat one; a management consultant must interview the client who seeks help. And these professionals cannot use their skills in advance of a patient or client requesting their services.

The pattern of consumption also differs. In the case of manufactured products, the consumer is free to determine the time and intensity of the use of the product purchased, be it a piano, an automobile, or a television set. In the absence of a breakdown requiring repair, it is the consumer's decision alone that determines the pattern of use. The situation is clearly different in the case of professional services: Even the hour of a marriage or a funeral will depend on the availability of the minister. The family that requires the presence of one must work out a mutually satisfactory time. Patients who seek early appointments with specialists, even if recommended by their personal physicians, may have to wait a fortnight or more if the latter have crowded schedules. The fact that the patient has the desire, a need, and the money to pay for the consultation is not determining; the provider's schedule controls.

The determinants of investment differ greatly as between manufacturing and professional services. In the former case, the owners, or management operating on their behalf, assess whether the outlook is favorable for using some part of their current profits (or contracting loans) to broaden or deepen the physical plant and equipment to produce additional units that can be sold at a price likely to cover the costs of the investment and something more. The investment structure for professional services is radically different. It involves a long-term commitment by the individual, some seven to ten or more years of study and training beyond graduation from high school. The costs to the students and their families in terms of outlays for tuition and living expenses, plus income foregone or lack of earnings because of study, may amount to $100,000 or even more per student, depending on the field. But there is a related investment cost, one that is underwritten largely by society in the form of public expenditures for college, university, and professional-school education and training. In the case of medicine, law, religion, research, and still other areas of professional work, there are additional expenditures, by government or philanthropy, or both, for the support of the institutions without which professionals cannot function: hospitals, the courts, churches, research laboratories. A much looser connection exists between the outlays for, and the rewards that accrue to, professionals and the private funds that entrepreneurs use to increase their income and wealth.

The employment patterns that characterize a manufacturing plant and a multispeciality medical practice or law firm also differ markedly. The proportions of professionals to support personnel are inverted. In the former case, relatively small numbers of professionals are used in direct production activities, although large numbers may be deployed in service functions, from finance to marketing. In professional practices, the critical work is performed by professionals, with assists from technical and secretarial staff. In manufacturing, the key to efficient production is the optimal balance between operators and machines; in professional practices the key is a two-pronged relation: between professionals and clients, and between nonprofessionals and professionals. Although there is some scope in the latter case for improved utilization involving the substitution of machines and paraprofessionals for professionals, the margins are relatively small.

The most striking contrast between goods and services relates to the system of social control. In the former instance, developed nations rely heavily on competition in the marketplace to assure that the consumer pays a price that yields only conventional, not monopoly, profits. In the realm of professional services, the state uses licensing as one way of assuring that professionals possess a stipulated level of knowledge and competence. Further, the state looks to the profession to take responsibility for preventing its members from exploiting the public and anticipates that the leadership will advance the boundaries of knowledge and technique. These instruments of social control do not replace, but rather modify, reliance on the marketplace, which still exercises considerable indirect influence on supply, allocation, and price.

To summarize the argument up to this point, the output of professional services differs from the conventional model used to explain the output of goods in the following major regards:

1. The criticality of educated and trained personnel in the production of services
2. The inability to produce for inventory and to ship professional services from one location to another
3. The necessity for consumers to interact directly with the provider in order to consume the service
4. The long-term investment that professionals-to-be must make in their preparation, and the concomitant heavy social investments that are required to enable them to obtain training and use their skills effectively
5. The severe limits to substituting either capital or less-trained personnel for professionals
6. The reliance on licensing and professional associations, rather than the market, to protect the consumer from exploitation

The thrust of this section is to call attention to some of the important ways in which the provision and purchase of health services differ from the conventional market relations that govern the production and distribution of goods. The plants used to produce the goods that business enterprises and the consumer need and are able to pay for are privately owned, and they will keep operating only so long as their capacity is required to meet the demand of the market and yield a profit to the owners. An unprofitable plant may be kept in operation for a year or two, or even a little longer, if the management anticipates that the demand and price will soon strengthen, but if their expectations are found wrong, closure and disinvestment will occur.

Hospitals, emergency rooms, and clinics are the principal locales where physicians provide services, together with their own offices. The vast majority of general hospital beds as well as emergency rooms and clinics are in nonprofit institutions built largely with philanthropic monies. The second largest component is governmental hospitals. Only a small percent-age, under 10 percent of all acute beds, and a much lower per-centage of emergency room and clinic visits, are in for-profit institutions. Without adducing evidence to support the proposi-tion, let me stipulate that the boards of trustees of voluntary hospitals and the administrators of great medical institutions do not use the same calculus in deciding whether or not to keep operating as do profit-seeking enterprises. This is not to say that they can keep their doors open indefinitely if their revenues fall below their expenditures over an extended period or if the legislative body cuts off their allocation. But market considerations do not predominate.

In terms of office practice, both with respect to the hours and intensity with which they work and the number of years they keep working, physicians are sensitive to economic considera-tions, including their desire for income and wealth, keeping an eye on the schedules of their colleagues. Even so, one cannot use a competitive pricing model to explain more than a small facet of their behavior, much of which reflects custom, tradi-tion, and personal preference.

Because the consumer of professional services must come in-to direct contact with the provider, if only by telephone, but frequently in person to permit a hands-on examination, the lo-cation of hospitals and physicians' offices is a matter of critical importance. To consider the latter matter first: "Getting to the site of care takes little time for most people. For about half of medically attended conditions, travel time was less than fif-teen minutes. For over four-fifths . . . people reached a place of care within a half-hour. Only 4.8 percent of the conditions re-quired journeys of forty-five minutes or longer" (Department of Health, Education and Welfare: 2). However, about one in five patients had to wait for an hour, and one in twelve, over two hours, before being treated.

When it comes to the distribution of acute hospital beds, and more particularly to the distribution of services that require specialized staff and equipment such as open heart surgery, co-balt therapy, or dialysis for end-stage renal disease, significant numbers of patients are poorly located for ready access. Secondary and tertiary centers of care cannot be established and maintained unless the adjacent area is sufficiently populated to command the time and talents of the providers. When people live in sparsely populated areas, they have to travel considerable distances for such specialized care. There is no more possibility of having a tertiary hospital every fifty miles than there is of having a major league baseball team or Broadway theater. The number of potential users is too small, the supply of talent too sparse. Goods can be shipped to the smallest hamlet, but in a free society physicians cannot be persuaded to establish practice in outlying areas, not even if they are guaranteed a reasonable income.

The consumption of health services requires the individual—or a surrogate in the case of children and the incompetent—to initiate the process. Not only must consumers take the first step, but after having made contact with providers they will profit from the encounter only if they follow the advice proffered, from going to surgeons to be operated on to taking medicine for infections. Unless patients initiate action when they first become aware of symptoms, as with bloody stools or nonhealing sores on the tongue, they may place themselves at serious risk, for the cancers may spread to the point where they can no longer be controlled. We also know from many studies that slippage in communication between patient and physician in either or both directions will result in less than optimal treatment. Since good medical care implies a long-term relationship between a patient who trusts the physician and a physician who obtains satisfaction from treating the patient, there is considerable opportunity for such slippage among patients who do not receive routine care from the same physician (about one in five) because they are uninterested or unable to establish such a relationship. The customer can buy a bottle of liquor by announcing a preferred brand and placing a bill on the counter. The patient seeking treatment for alcoholism confronts a much more complex transaction.

The pattern of investment differs in manufacturing and in health care delivery. In the former instance, society pays for young people to acquire basic competencies in the publicly financed school system, but the factory that turns out the product is responsible for the specific training of its work force. Not so in the case of professional services. Here society covers most of the expenditures involved in the higher education and professional training of future practitioners—as well as paying, in the case of physicians, for the costly workplace, the hospital.

One of the outstanding differences between the production of goods and professional services relates to the conditions of employment. In a manufacturing enterprise, employers attract and retain workers by offering them wages and other benefits that are equal or superior to the offers of competing employers. Once having hired them, an employer is more or less free to decide how to deploy them, something that is done with an eye to optimizing their contribution to the total output. In the case of the professions, the state, through licensing, stipulates the assignments that different groups of workers are permitted or not permitted to do, reserving to the fully qualified professional the broadest scope of action. With the imprimatur of the state, physicians are able to determine the allocation of work among health providers and in so doing are able to capture a large part of the rewards. Some forms of therapy, such as psychotherapy, are more or less uncontrolled—any person can offer advice and counsel—but most active interventions, from prescribing drugs to treating specific organs, are seriously circumscribed by statute and administrative regulation.

Although it is an oversimplification to see the market controlling the output of goods and nonmarket arrangements, such as licensing of physicians and community planning for hospitals, dominating the delivery of health services, the gross distinction has merit. While there are important social controls other than the market impacting the production of goods, from variances for construction to Office of Economic Opportunity regulations, and while there are elements of price competition both among medical practitioners and among hospitals, the fact remains that the two sectors—goods and service production—respond to a different set of incentives and rewards.

This review of the characteristics of health services production and distribution has called attention to the following important characteristics:

1. The principal institutions providing health care services do not operate on the basis of a profit-seeking model.
2. The distribution of health care services involves face-to-face relations between providers and purchasers.

3. The high order of specialization implies that many consumers will be forced to travel substantial distances from their homes to obtain such service.
4. Consumers of health care services must initiate action, and the extent to which they will profit will depend in considerable measure on the continuity and quality of the interactions between their physicians and themselves.
5. Society is the principal investor in the education and training of health professionals and in providing the workplace.
6. Government determines through licensing what different groups of medical personnel are permitted to do and, in the process, establishes the physician in the dominant role.
7. Policing, rather than the market, is the principal instrument of social control in the health care industry.

Among many groups, a high degree of restiveness exists today concerning the present circumstances and future prospects of American medicine in relation to the general welfare. Total outlays for health care are too large, considering that additional expenditures appear to contribute little to the reduction of morbidity and mortality. The rate of increase in health care prices, at half again above the average for all prices, is deflecting too much of the consumer's restricted purchasing power into the health care industry, a trend that cannot long continue without serious social consequences. The entire system is skewed in the direction of therapy rather than prevention, and the quality of care leaves much to be desired. Current incentives draw people for treatment into the hospital rather than into ambulatory settings that would be less costly, and there are no effective mechanisms to avoid duplication and underutilization of facilities. Physicians are able to assure themselves of unjustifiably high incomes. Insurance, with no, or only small, deductibles encourages overutilization; reimbursement procedures encourage hospitals to be wasteful; and the quality and reach of hospital insurance is inadequate in the case of catastrophic illness. Many low-income people face serious difficulties in obtaining necessary services, and the structure of health care for the aged, especially the feeble aged, is seriously deficient.

Three principal responses have been advanced to cope with these shortcomings: controls, competition, and voluntarism, each reflecting a distinctive ideology. Those who advocate a stronger system of controls by means of national health insurance believe that such an approach will assure better coverage of the population and at the same time constrain total outlays. The advocates of competition look to the multiplication of new structures for delivering health care (health maintenance organizations—HMOs), greater reliance on coinsurance and deductibles, and more consumer choice. They have faith in the allocative efficiency of the market, if only it is permitted to operate. The voluntarists read the record differently. They acknowledge many of the shortcomings, especially the unchecked inflation, but they are impressed with the flexibility of the health care system and its accomplishments and oppose broad restructuring, believing that such an effort will destroy much that is good in exchange for gains that remain putative.

How does the preceding analysis of professional services in general, and health services in particular, relate to our present discontent and our goals for a strengthened health care system at the end of the century? Our answers must be focused on the realities of service output, distribution, and consumption rather than on general principles or specific mechanisms that attract philosophers, economists, and ideologists. To provide perspective, it may be useful to consider briefly the principal transforming agents that altered in substantial degree, and largely for the better, the structuring and functioning of American medicine in the past half-century. Without ascribing significance to the ordering of the factors, I would single out the following:

1. The maintenance and expansion of a strong medical education structure that was able to attract, educate, and indoctrinate young people in the science and art of providing health care at the same time that the medical schools broadened and deepened the knowledge pool through new research.

2. The increasing sophistication of the nation's hospitals, particularly those with teaching programs, which provided an environment conducive to treating the sick and injured

under preferred conditions in which multiple specialists working with paramedical personnel were able to provide a much improved level of care.

3. The substantial gains in commercial and nonprofit insurance carriers, which created the market whereby people of modest income could protect themselves against the extraordinary expenses of hospitalized illnesses.

4. Major governmental investments, both state and federal, directed to increasing the supplies of health personnel and health facilities, the liberal funding of research, financing care for specified categories of patients, and putting into place various planning and control mechanisms.

5. Finally, the strong response of the American people to the potentialities of modern medicine as reflected in their support as consumers, purchasers of insurance, taxpayers, and voluntary contributors. Ivan Illich and his colleagues have made little headway in their efforts to convince the American people that modern medicine is dysfunctional. The public has voted with its feet, its head, its heart, and its purse to affirm its liberal support for modern medical care.

The remainder of this presentation is directed to specifying the underlying sources of strength of the extant system and the costly consequences that would follow upon reforms that deliberately or inadvertently undermined these sources. Our attention will be riveted on the dynamics of professional services— how they are produced, distributed, and consumed. Because of the inability to foresee the secondary consequences of new societal interventions, any attempt at reform that ignores these dynamics is certain to fail, and even a high sensitivity to them will not guarantee success. I will consider sequentially professional manpower, innovations, intermediaries, government, and the consuming public as the critical elements that can affect for better or worse the condition of American medicine in the years to come. But what follows is only half the story. It focuses on what our emerging understanding of services suggests should *not* be done. The second part, which will concentrate on what needs doing, must await further analytic work on the theory of services and the institutional framework that will prevail.

Medicine has long been an attractive profession to a large number of the college-educated, who have opted for it because of its career opportunities, intellectual challenge, and working conditions. The number of well-qualified young people applying for admission to U.S. medical schools has always exceeded the number of places available. The willingness of young people to work very hard to gain admission to medical school, to continue working very hard to acquire specialty certification, and, in addition, to work very hard after starting practice reflects the synergistic relations among the challenge of the work, the competition for prestige and status, and the fact that the level of their income is closely linked to the hours they work.

In recent years, as a result of the increasing coverage by third-party payers, several new trends have emerged: Physicians' incomes are relatively close to an all-time high since physicians no longer do any, or at best only a small amount of, "free work" either in hospital or out. On the other hand, the paperwork connected with their billings, the pressures to control their fees, the threat of malpractice suits, and the constraints on their freedom of decision (professional standards review organizations—PSROs—and second opinions in surgery) are steadily eroding one of the major attractions that medicine long offered—a high degree of freedom to practice according to one's own lights.

There are many among the reformers who believe that the aforementioned attempts to control physicians' incomes and modes of practice have not gone far enough. They see little point in permitting physicians to continue to earn four times the average wage; they see less point in having society subsidize the costs of medical education without getting any service in return. Hence they look with favor on the National Health Service Corps as a way of solving two problems at once: getting a return from physicians whose education was subsidized by requiring them to practice in underserved areas, on the basis of one year of service for every year of subsidy.

As is true of so many societal arrangements, a reasonable proposal is not the same as an effective solution. Consider such a reasonable proposal as one aimed at reducing the "high" incomes of physicians by requiring them to justify their judgments when they differ from the norm (utilization review), or one that interdicts their ability to take joint action against potential interlopers (antitrust), or that otherwise circumscribes their freedom to act (recertification). But acting on all of these fronts, and still others, is by no means fail-safe. The key to the quality of professional services is the continued commitment of the professional, a condition that social intervention can destroy but that it is poorly positioned to create.

Freedom, income, hours of work, and commitment are critical determinants of how professionals act and react. The more constricted their freedom and the more their income depends on meeting formal criteria, the fewer their hours of work and the less their commitment. How can it be otherwise? If physicians are forced to follow established therapeutic regimens, they have little incentive to explore and reflect, to assume added responsibilities. If they are paid the same for doing more or less, they are likely to opt for the easier life.

There is a related aspect of the social control of professional services that must not be overlooked. Professionals, by definition (and often, as in the case of physicians, by law), possess knowledge and control techniques that they share with no other group. Hence it is difficult, and some would say impossible, for government to control the behavior of professionals. Some might reply, not so, for government can use professionals to control professionals. Up to a point this may be true, but only up to a point, because the more distinguished and able members of a profession are unlikely to enter into a position, much less remain in one, that places them in continuing conflict with their peers.

What is the burden of these observations for the health care system in the years ahead? First, the steady inroads of the bureaucratization of medicine on the freedom of physicians should neither be ignored nor minimized. They hold a serious threat to the future vitality of American medicine. The threat is that much greater because of several adverse developments on the economic front: The steeply rising costs of obtaining a medical education; the determination of the federal government to secure required services for subsidies advanced; the certain rapid rise in the total number of physicians per 100,000 population, three times greater in the 1980s than in the preceding quarter century, which will inevitably tend to reduce the relative incomes of physicians, however much it will contribute to increasing total costs; and the continuing efforts—of uncertain effectiveness—of third-party payers to moderate the rise in physician fees.

There is no need to accuse the medical profession of being excessively concerned with material rewards in order to emphasize that the foregoing confluence of events will of itself reduce the attractiveness of the profession. Hence, social interventions likely to further weaken the profession should be carefully weighed against putative gains, for it would not take a great deal of additional pressure to undermine seriously the morale of physicians to a point where their orientation to a high level of professional accomplishment is permanently weakened.

Easy access to enlarged funding for education, research, hospital care, in fact for almost every aspect of health care, in the third quarter of this century sustained a high level of innovation. Medical schools were able to broaden and deepen their faculty resources, laboratories, and curricula. Even though an occasional critic might take umbrage at some of these developments, arguing that the newly won domination of the research-oriented professors carried an important hidden cost by downplaying clinical excellence, most observers would read the record favorably. The same holds for the strong push toward specialization, in which the teaching hospital played such a critical role. Here the level of criticism rises a little higher because of the popularization of the idea that the nation moved too far in the direction of specialization, leaving the public with an insufficient number of primary-care physicians. The evidence simply does not sustain the latter claim, and nobody has come forward to prove that physicians who have less training and who devote themselves exclusively to first-encounter medicine will find such a career rewarding professionally or will be sought out by large numbers of the public. The best that one can say for the critics of specialization—and I am not inclined to give them the benefit of the doubt—is that they have failed to prove their case.

In the mid-1960s, discerning that the many claims of soon-to-be-achieved significant breakthroughs (cancer, heart disease, rheumatism) that medical researchers had made when they advocated larger funding had not been realized, the federal government moved to expand access to the existing health care system, primarily through Medicare and Medicaid. Within a decade, federal expenditures for health increased about tenfold, but by the end of this period it was increasingly clear that the cutting edge of the health system—the medical schools, the research establishment, and the teaching hospitals—were hard put to it to maintain, much less expand, their level of operations. This is what I have called the Shannon paradox, because Dr. James Shannon of the National Institutes of Health was, to my knowledge, the first to point out that steeply rising total expenditures, reflecting the imperatives of more services, could be associated with stagnation and decline at the frontiers.

The combination of a society seeking to expand access for underserved populations and at the same time to improve the quantity and quality of the services to the entire population, with the simultaneous effort to constrain total expenditures, casts an ominous shadow ahead for institutions at the cutting edge. Just consider the recent reductions in the federal government's capitation payments or subsidies for medical schools, the continuing tightness in the budgets of the National Institutes of Health, and the pressures being exerted by state rate-making authorities, which are rapidly eroding the endowments of leading teaching hospitals by providing below-cost reimbursement. Any effort to centralize the funding for the health care industry should be assessed for its likely impact on innovation. In my view it is likely to have a disastrous effect.

The long delay in seriously debating, much less passing, national health insurance has had the advantage of giving both the advocates and the opponents time to probe more deeply into our own experience and that of foreign countries. In 1980 no responsible group is any longer advocating a national health system in which the federal government not only would be the sole source of funding but would exercise direct operational control over the entire system, as in the case of the National Health Service in the United Kingdom. Part of the explanation for this backing away from sole reliance on the federal government bespeaks the considerable success of commercial and nonprofit insurance carriers in providing reasonable coverage for costly medical care for the majority of the population. Part of the explanation indicates the growing skepticism of the public about the ability of government to deliver on its promises. While few have read the MEGA report, prepared at the request of Secretary Richardson when he was head of Health, Education, and Welfare, the American public has intuitively come to appreciate that even statutory promises are no guarantee of their securing access to services to which they are entitled, certainly not to services of desirable quality. The MEGA report revealed that the gap between the numbers entitled to services and the numbers receiving them was on the order of one to four.

There are three intermediaries that should be assessed in terms of the future direction of the health care industry: insurance carriers; HMOs and other new structures for the delivery of care; and planning and control mechanisms, from state rate authorities to Health Systems Agencies (HSAs).

With respect to the commercial insurance carriers, one can note a belated interest and concern on their part to play a more active role, from subsidizing new forms of delivery of care to utilizing their considerable leverage to help contain costs. Since these profit-seeking companies and their nonprofit allies are aware of the growing concern of the public and government (both federal and state) to move in the direction of better services at lower costs, they have come to appreciate that they must undertake a more active part, for their continued inaction is an invitation to government to fill the breach. The commercial carriers defined their role as middlemen during the past decades, authenticating claims and paying out money to beneficiaries and to providers without becoming deeply involved in efforts directed to assuring a more effective use of the health dollars over which they had discretion. At most, they sought to avoid being victimized by claimants who engaged in fraud or providers who submitted inflated bills.

Blue Cross and Blue Shield have been charged, and with considerable justification, with a related failing that resulted from their being so closely aligned with providers—hospitals and physicians. The Plans have been criticized for not exerting leverage to eliminate the waste that arises from the duplication of beds and services and for not encouraging providers to experiment with new and improved forms of health care delivery. The most serious charges center on their writing policies primarily for inpatient treatment and for first-dollar coverage, which together contributed significantly to cost acceleration.

No institution that is doing well looks for trouble, and both commercial and nonprofit health care insurers for a long time enjoyed the rewards of profits and growth by avoiding confrontations with the medical and hospital establishments with whom they were so intimately bound. In thinking ahead about the changes that are likely to occur, one of the more important, but problematic, forecasts is the future behavior of the health insurance sector. One formulation follows: The extent to which government becomes more directly involved in every aspect of health care, beyond its increasing role as financier, will depend in large measure on the innovative capacities of the insurance intermediaries and their capacity to respond to old and new challenges, from cost containment to home care. The contention, advanced by Alain Enthoven and others, that the insurers have been remiss in not offering a wider range of policies with deductibles and coinsurance features appears to me to be largely beside· the point in light of the tremendous growth in recent years of major-medical policies. Moreover, the insurers are not responsible for the trade unionists' intransigence with respect to first-dollar coverage. A more valid criticism would be directed to the slowness with which the insurers have experimented with comprehensive coverage, ambulatory as well as inpatient.

We are about one decade into the era that looked to HMOs to be the great innovator in health care. There are many explanations and excuses for their modest growth, as well as for the modest growth of other forms of physicians' cooperatives aimed at providing comprehensive care at affordable prices. There are those who keep the faith and who still expect that by the end of the century these new delivery systems will account for a majority of the health services delivered to the American people. They may turn out to be right, but the odds are against them because of the entrepreneurial and managerial talents required to establish and maintain these cooperatives, which confront additional hurdles in that many

physicians are loath to circumscribe their freedom to practice
and many middle-class consumers are disinclined to restrict
their freedom of choice. If the key to professional services, as
we have argued, is the interaction between provider and consumer, it is difficult to see how modest dollar savings will lead
many purchasers to restrict their freedom of choice voluntarily. We will probably have a sufficient number of new forms of
delivery, moderated by broadened and deepened insurance coverage, to satisfy those who are disenchanted with the present
structure of solo or group fee-for-service. But it would take a
zealot to see HMOs and their offspring and relations transforming the delivery of health care by this century's end. More
consumer choice in the areas of health insurance and delivery
systems predicated on intensified competition among providers
is likely to prove chimerical because of resistance from providers and the skepticism of consumers. Therefore, the logical
next question is the outlook for planning and control mechanisms at federal, state, and areal levels.

The federal government, by turning the appropriations spig-
ot on and off, has had a considerable impact on facility construction, the production of health manpower, the
encouragement of biomedical research, the broadening of access for the poor and the aged, the expansion of new programs
(from renal dialysis to emergency medical care), and in still
other regards. But its effect on the system other than through
the expenditure route has been slight. It has had limited or
almost no success in redistributing health resources to underserved areas; the PSRO effort, according to a recent report of
the Congressional Budget Office, has yet to justify itself; little
or no progress has been made to squeeze out the acknowledged
surplus of acute hospital beds, variously calculated as between
10 and 15 percent of the total; and regionalization is proceeding at a snail's pace.

Spurred and financed by the federal government, planning
at the state level is making uneven progress, but in a minority
of states, including such important ones as New York, Massachusetts, California, and Pennsylvania, one can point to significant advances in state actions directed to influencing
facilities, manpower, services, and rates. Some believe that
these efforts are doomed to frustration and failure; they see the

controllers being captured sooner rather than later by those whom they are seeking to control. That is a possible, but by no means a certain, outcome. For better or worse, because of what economists define as natural monopolies, power companies, telephone companies, and broadcasting companies have not been set loose to compete with no holds barred. Under special conditions of technology, the market, and the structure of production, untrammeled competition leads not to the efficient use of resources and lower prices but to the opposite—a waste in resources and higher prices. The question is whether complex institutions like hospitals, particularly hospitals providing secondary and tertiary care, should be permitted or encouraged to enter into unrestrained competition. The presumption is that such an approach might yield the following dysfunctional results: Inadequate coverage for vulnerable areas and population groups that lack the capacity to raise the required capital sums through philanthropy, and where many patients just above the Medicaid cutoff point are unable to pay more than part of their bills; the absence of adequate standby capacity to treat emergency cases (accident victims); the high probability that the total bed capacity would shrink to a point where long queues would exacerbate waiting time for admission for inpatient treatment; the shrinkage of facilities to treat ambulatory patients as more and more hospitals would be forced to close their doors; the seriously adverse effects on the practice of medicine resulting from the loss of hospital staff affiliations of many physicians. Such adverse effects, even if they would not be universal, have a sufficiently high probability to advise against recourse to competition as the preferred regulator of the hospital market.

The Health Planning Act of 1974, after giving a piece of the action to the federal government and another piece to state governments, threw its weight back of the creation of a regional capability named the Health Systems Agency. As a major designer of the act remarked, to plan without having resources to back up one's decision is to plan in a vacuum. The HSAs do not even have the resources to staff themselves adequately or to obtain and analyze the data out of which their plans should be shaped. The typical HSA suffers further limitations: No party that finds itself in opposition to a recommendation is likely to acquiesce unless forced to by higher authority. And higher authorities (state agencies) are careful not to make unnecessary waves for their political bosses. Moreover, the aggrieved party has resort to the courts.

If the United States is to make better and more effective use of its multihundred-billion-dollar investment in health care in meeting the priority health needs of its people, it has no option but to strengthen its planning capabilities at every level, but especially locally. It is here that people live and it is here that they seek access to providers in clinics, offices, and hospitals. Their prospect of getting more and better care will depend largely on how well the leadership in their community, professional and lay, succeeds in recapturing the underutilized and unused resources and redeploying them and in directing new resources to priority needs. There is nothing easy in such arrangements, but only the naive believe that significant health reform is easy.

One of the critical facets of the current debate about alternative approaches to health reform, as well as one of the crucial determinants of the shape of the system in the year 2000, focuses on the potentiality and limitations of government to affect structure and outcome. For clarity, one should distinguish the following: Government as financier, deliverer of services, and controller; and the distinctions between the federal government and lower levels of government (state and local).

The record of government as financier points to the following: The federal and state governments, acting in loose cooperation in the post-World War II period, were able to increase substantially the flow of resources into the health industry through new hospital construction, the expansion of health training institutions, and the broadening access of the poor and the aged to health services achieved by substituting tax for consumer dollars. In addition, one must note federal support for biomedical research and expensive new service programs such as treatment of end-stage renal disease.

It would be a grievous error, however, to project this steeply rising expenditure trend forward into the last two decades of this century. All the signs point in the opposite direction—the flattening in real terms of expenditures for research; the early removal of the 2 percent override for hospitals under Medicare;

the strenuous efforts of the Carter administration to put a ceiling on allowable increases in hospital costs; and the actions of many state legislatures to cut back on their Medicaid outlays.

A reasonable formulation of government as financier would be as follows: In periods of budgetary ease, governments can increase substantially the flow of resources into the health care industry and in the process expand the capacity of the system to deliver a broader range of services to more people. But the strategic position of providers, particularly medical schools, hospitals, and physicians, to deflect a considerable part of the additional resources to their own purposes implies a high ratio of new dollars for each increment of additional output. Gains to the consuming public do not come cheaply.

When one shifts the focus from government as financier to government as provider of services, the tale goes something like this: Governments have difficulty in providing direct health services to the poor, the mentally ill, and special population groups such as veterans, native Americans, and inmates of prisons, because of the problems in attracting physicians and other health personnel, who generally can find more interesting and lucrative work in the nongovernmental sector. As a consequence, most governmentally owned and operated health facilities provide an inferior level of care. To the extent that such medical installations are operated by state and local governments, which are more severely constrained financially than the federal government, the level of service leaves even more to be desired.

There is a danger in politicians' and reformers' promising to deliver more and better care to the American people without being forced to confront this issue of the unfavorable record of government as a direct provider of health services. True, the starry-eyed might reply that the past need not repeat itself. If the federal government assumed responsibility for organizing and running a National Health Service, as in the United Kingdom, it would no longer be forced to compete in the market and would be better positioned to deliver on its promises. But such a reply simply shifts the argument from the known into the unknown. What is meant by saying that the federal government will "organize and operate" the health service for all Americans? There is nothing in the past performance of the federal government that would give one confidence in its ability to deliver an increased quantity and quality of such services. The odds favor serious slippage, not improvement. And, in any case, as noted earlier, no serious politician is now advocating such a fundamental reform.

This brings us to the third and last dimension of government's role in health care—that of controller. Here the record is mixed. The several levels of government have performed various functions, from public health enforcement to the outlawing of dangerous substances in food and drugs, with considerable success, although there are conservative critics who believe that the hidden costs of such enforcement come too high in terms of hamstringing the pharmaceutical companies in financing innovations, and there are environmental critics who rail against the laxness in government's controlling of carcinogenic factors. But the subtleties of cost-benefit analysis to one side, the standard-setting and enforcement activities of government in the arena of health care can probably be rated as fair, possibly higher.

When it comes to the heartland of health care—controlling the actions of hospitals and medical practitioners—the record of government is equivocal. The optimists would say that government has acted sensibly to proceed with a light hand, leaving most of the controlling to professional societies, from the Joint Commission on Accreditation of Hospitals to the state and county medical societies and the specialty boards. It is better, in this view, for professionals to set the standards and to enforce them. But the critics disagree, some strenuously. They point to a long list of abuses that the professional bodies fail to pick up and, worse still, fail to correct once they become cognizant of them.

It is hard to disagree with the criticism that professional societies have been lax in using their powers to discipline malfeasants. But the remedy is not obvious. A larger number of the governmental officials—especially the nonphysicians—who are engaged to police the industry may not prove efficient or effective. The preferred alternative may be to apply additional societal pressures to encourage professional groups to take their controlling obligations more seriously and to discharge them more effectively.

There is another aspect of the control function that warrants attention because of its potential influence on both federal and state actions in the health arena. The courts, administrative agencies such as the Department of Health and Human Services (HHS) and the Federal Trade Commission, and Congress, through subsidies for HMOs, are seeking to broaden the role of competition in the health care market by providing more choice for consumers and reduced opportunities for providers to make monopolistic gains. But at the same time, both federal and state governments are moving along a second track of influencing resource allocations, prices, and outputs through administrative rule and regulations, by employing instrumentalities such as rate commissions and health services area–planning organizations.

The proponents of the market approach argue that market competition is the best and most effective regulator and that governments would be well advised to further its scale and scope. Hence their advice is to eliminate perverse incentives and rewards such as the current use of tax subsidies to increase the demand for hospital insurance by reducing its true cost to the purchaser, which in time encourages physicians to use more costly services than they would otherwise resort to. The advocates of greater competition look to the establishment and expansion of new delivery systems, particularly HMOs and their variants, which stress comprehensive prepayment with a tilt toward ambulatory over inpatient care as a source of large savings. But the fact that HMOs, even with federal subsidies, have made slow gains suggests that their financial advantages are not all that evident or convincing.

Because governments remain uncertain about the ability of competition to assure cost effectiveness and cost containment, they are proceeding along parallel lines to improve their planning and control mechanisms to accomplish the following: to limit the total inflow of resources into the health care system; to improve the allocation of such resources so as to provide adequate coverage for the entire population without tolerating the continued underutilization of resources; to provide reimbursement plans that will encourage hospitals to economize in the use of additional resources, thereby dampening the rate of inflation; to establish fee schedules that provide physicians with a reasonable, but not excessive, return for the services they render patients for whom government is financially responsible; and to rationalize the facilities structure to provide a balance among the different types of treatment beds, from tertiary hospitals to supervised living arrangements for the feeble aged.

The enumeration of these complex objectives underscores the wide gap between the extant legislative, administrative, and planning mechanisms and the capacity of these mechanisms to perform effectively. Those who are skeptical about the capacity of government are inclined to write off this approach, which is in an early stage of development. But if the foregoing strictures about the inherent limitations of relying on competition are apposite, the ineluctable conclusion emerges that the health care system cannot be brought under effective social control. However, that appears to be both premature and presumptuous. A democracy is entitled to more time for experimentation before such a pessimistic conclusion is accepted.

We now come to a consideration of the last of the key actors, the role of consumers of health services and how their behavior, individually and collectively, may help to reshape the health care system in the decades ahead. We noted earlier that consumers are a critical element in the provision of all health care services: They must initiate action; they must interact with and respond to the recommendations of physicians; it is up to them to follow the regimens that the physicians prescribe and to report back on any untoward results that may develop. They must take action to protect their health by following sensible diets, avoiding excesses, and engaging in regular exercise. In recent years, through law and administrative action, the consumers have come to play a much larger role in the decisionmaking process, since medical intervention involves an admixture of potential benefits and risks. They must be consulted about undergoing surgery, about entering on series of drug treatments with possible adverse side effects, and about agreeing to life-prolonging procedures in the event of terminal illness.

The decades immediately following World War II captured the imagination of the American people: They had great faith and trust in the curative powers of specialized medicine. Of all the forces leading to the rapid growth and development of the health care system, none was more potent than consumer enthusiasm. But we may be entering a new era, one in which the public can distinguish among the conditions for which medicine has useful answers; those where it can make a contribution but for which it has no cure; and the large number of conditions where medicine may be able to prolong life for a brief period but is impotent to reverse the natural history of the disease. To the extent that the public becomes more sophisticated and makes such discriminations, we may find consumers no longer willing to undergo radical interventions, surgical and other, in their last year of life. Further, many of those in the higher age groups will distinguish the chronic disabilities with which they will have to contend as best they can through their own resources and with the help of family and friends, and those where medical intervention may have something to offer them.

There is a second arena in which the consumer is more involved. Consider the partial success of antismoking campaigns, improved nutrition, greater participation in systematic exercise, and other health maintenance activities. It would be misleading to argue that modern societies should redirect their efforts from curative to preventive medicine: We simply do not know how to prevent many of the worst diseases and accidents that afflict modern men and women. But it is correct to involve the public more actively in the maintenance of its own health. With six out of seven young Americans graduating from high school and more than one out of four from college, the scope for participation in their own health maintenance and therapy is substantially greater than it was in the past when the society had only a small percentage of educated persons.

There remain additional functions in which the changing behavior of the consumer, acting collectively, may be able to make a difference. The great nonprofit hospital system in the United States owes much to the leaders of philanthropy; the growth of nonprofit Blue Cross and Blue Shield Plans involved at least some representatives of the public, although the decisionmaking power remained for the most part in the hands of health professionals and their managerial cadres. Recent changes at neighborhood, area, state, and federal levels have seen the substantially enlarged participation of public representatives in various health-planning and policymaking bodies. The sophisticated observer might argue that the public representatives are window dressing, little more, and that effective decisionmaking power remains in the hands of health professionals. But such a judgment, projected into the future, is too gross. Professionals will inevitably continue to be critical decisionmakers involving the delivery of health care, about which they know more then the rest of the citizenry. But the consumers, who pay for the services directly through insurance or as taxpayers, clearly must be heard, their criticisms heeded, their recommendations considered. Since the greater involvement of consumer groups in the health care process is of recent date, it would be premature to conclude that the whole effort is a public-relations gimmick.

In brief recapitulation of the five critical dimensions of health care as they affect the general welfare:

1. Serious threats on the horizon suggest that the practice of medicine may no longer be as attractive a career as in the past, with significantly adverse consequences for the quality of health care available to the American people.
2. A shortage of funding for innovation, medical education, research, and teaching hospitals could severely retard the future progress of medical care.
3. Of the three intermediaries, insurance carriers, HMOs, and planning mechanisms, the first is strong and largely effective; the second and third must still prove themselves.
4. Government as financier has been able to play a key role in expanding the health care industry. Government as direct provider of services and as controller of the industry has been much less successful.
5. Consumers as individuals have a larger role to play in the future in the maintenance of their own health and as active parties in restoring it; and together they will insist on having more say in transforming the system so as to provide themselves with more benefits.

It would be easy for the reader to interpret the foregoing as a defense of the status quo, as a plea for keeping the present system intact, for assuring that physicians remain at the helm.

Justification for this interpretation is strengthened when one recalls that the analysis argued explicitly about the dangers of a reduction in the relative earnings of physicians, about the limited capacity of prepayment plans to grow, and about the likelihood that national health insurance, if passed, would lead to promises that could not be met. And if the foregoing were not warning enough against current approaches to restructure the health care industry, one can point to the deep pessimism expressed about the "in doctrine" that deregulation and competition can assure the future efficiency and effectiveness of the health care system.

I have raised the flag to warn the inexperienced sailor that the seas are strong and that he should proceed cautiously. But that does not imply that we should fail to become engaged. In fact, in a dynamic economy and society, disengagement can be the most dangerous of all stances, for those standing cautiously on the sidelines are likely to be pushed aside by others who know, or think they know, where they are headed and are pressing full steam ahead. Those who believe, as I do, that the present system has more to commend it than to fault it have no option but to consider each of the major criticisms that are being leveled against it and to suggest the directions for remedial action that promise more gain than loss. But the one thing they dare not do is to adopt a head-in-the-sand approach.

There is little point in my dealing with the details of possible reforms. A more apposite approach will be for me to identify the critical issues that must be addressed and to suggest the bounds within which responsive actions should be undertaken. If the right issues are identified and if the goals are set forth correctly, the details can be left to later negotiations in the political and public arenas. At least this is the way that I plan to proceed.

Current criticisms about the role of the physician cover a wide range, including excessive earnings, inadequate self-policing, a preference for specialized over primary-care practice, efforts to engage in unfair practices to maintain a monopoly, a tendency to rely excessively on heroic interventions, a failure to engage patients in critical decisions affecting the possible outcome of therapy, and still other major, not to mention minor, complaints.

With physicians accounting for about 25 percent of all health care expenditures—second only to the costs of hospitalization—there are clearly good reasons for concern about the level and trend in their earnings. In terms of total expenditures, it is difficult to see how the trend can fail to move upward in the face of the large increases in numbers about to enter the profession. In terms of relative annual earnings, one must assume that the trend will be down, even if one believes, as I do, that physicians have some scope to influence their earnings by encouraging return visits.

There is also ground for concern about the other points of criticism outlined above. Clearly, a democratic society is entitled to intervene when it concludes that the privileges it has granted a professional group are not producing optimal social results, either because of abuse, neglect, self-interest, or any combination of these, and for still other reasons. But the challenge that a society faces when it decides to intervene involves the questions of which shortcomings, with which approaches, and in what sequence.

The boundary issues with respect to influencing the behavior of the individual physician and the medical profession appear to me to encompass the following: American medicine has long attracted substantial numbers of able young people who were willing to undergo a rigorous education and later to work hard because of the career rewards, monetary and nonmonetary. Among the most attractive career inducements was the substantial degree of freedom that the physician had to practice medicine according to his own best judgment, influenced, but not dictated to, by his peers. A society that is concerned that there is much wrong with its health care system, and that sees the physician as an individual and as a member of a profession responsible for the shortcomings of that system, runs the risk of intervening on so many fronts, from controlling residencies to controlling therapeutic regimens, that it might tip the career outcomes from highly positive to neutral or even negative. If that occurred, the future of medicine would no longer attract a large number of dedicated and committed professionals but would tilt the system in the direction of salaried workers who were willing to accept a trade of less responsibility and less income for a lower order of commitment and fewer hours of work. In my view, the American people would be the losers from such a trade.

When it comes to collective action on the part of physicians, the citizenry must seek new structures and new ways of interacting with the leaders of the profession. The political arena represents one stage where such interaction has taken place, and that will probably be even more crowded in the future. But in the pluralism that has been one of the nation's great strengths, other arenas should be explored where such interactions can be introduced or improved, from manpower planning to consumer complaints. It is no longer practical nor desirable to leave physicians in untrammeled control of the health care system. The citizenry has too large a stake in its future. But considerable experimentation will be needed before useful decisionmaking structures are built where leaders of the profession, along with representatives of the public, will be able to address jointly the options for strengthening the health care system and initiating actions to accomplish agreed upon goals.

There is a chorus of voices from government officials, voluntary health organizations, economists, consumer groups, organized labor, and employers, all addressing the need for action to contain the rapid rise in health expenditures. The preferred remedies range from the proposed federally legislated hospital reimbursement ceiling to voluntary action by hospitals. More extreme recommendations are aimed at altering the tax benefits that involve the purchase of health insurance in order to reflect its true cost and at establishing national health insurance, which would allocate an annual sum to be divided among providers. Some look to a checkrein on total expenditures, others to a restructuring of the delivery systems to substitute less- for more-expensive therapies. Still others favor a squeezing out of underutilized beds and services, both of which swell costs. The PSRO approach, now in its seventh year, has sought to contribute to cost containment by tightening the systems governing admission to, and length of stay in,. hospitals, but the most recent Congressional Budget Office review suggests that the approach has so far had little impact and is probably not going to have much in the future.

It is my considered opinion that there is no single or preferred way to control costs unless the American people agree to forego a great many benefits, including the advantages that flow from a mixed system of financing and operating its health care institutions. Does this mean that the public is powerless to slow the cost acceleration that has occurred? Far from it. First, it should be noted that the ever-increasing concern of the public with health cost inflation has led to the institution of various authorities and mechanisms, which are still in a formative stage but not so new as to be devoid of results. Several states can point to some success in slowing their costs. The engagement of the purchasers of insurance, particularly large employers and large trade unions, points to some prospective constraints from their side. Both nonprofit and commercial insurance carriers are becoming more actively involved. They recognize that they cannot keep acting solely as money conduits.

The old adage may fit—I don't claim it does—that by the time the public becomes aroused the issue is already on the way to solution. But more needs to be done, and that more requires political leadership, administrative sophistication, and community involvement. There are substantial margins for cost containment and quality improvement to be achieved from successful efforts at improved regionalization. At present, the nation not only has too many underutilized hospital beds, which add substantially to total outlays (possibly as much as $10 billion a year), but alongside these excess beds are expensive specialized services, from renal dialysis to cobalt treatments, many of which operate far below their optimum, which results both in higher costs and inferior quality. Admittedly, there is no easy way to make progress, much less fast progress, in moving to a higher degree of regionalization so that there would be enough, but not too many, institutions capable of providing these sophisticated services. One point of leadership ought to be the federal government; in the case of renal dialysis, it is the principal, and now almost the sole, financier of the service. The capacity of the federal government to take constructive action in this arena should be a touchstone of its capacity to assume a leadership role in rationalizing the health care industry. If it cannot initiate constructive actions to affect this single treatment mode, where it pays almost all the costs, it would be foolish to expect it to perform in other arenas where the problems are much more complex because of the involvement of many more principals, from state governments to private insurance companies.

Since Congress and the administration are able to intervene only if the groups supporting intervention are more powerful than those blocking it, and since there are small but potent groups that benefit from the present loose structure of federal expenditures for renal dialysis, the critical question here, and elsewhere, is whether leadership groups in the private sector, from nephrologists to insurance and hospital associations, will create the consensus without which the federal officials will be unable to act. Renal dialysis is no more than one illustration of where action is needed but where it must wait on a prior consensus from groups that are concerned about both costs and quality. The extent to which opportunities are translated into accomplishments through joint action will largely determine the quality of health care that will be available to the American people in the year 2000.

Some years ago, various groups interested in the reform of the health care system began to agitate in favor of placing representatives of consumers on various decisionmaking bodies, from hospital boards of trustees to the boards of directors of nonprofit insurance carriers. In the absence of any definitive study of this impetus, one is forced to impressionistic judgments. In my view, most of the effort to push consumer responsibilities to the fore was more symbolic than real. In only isolated cases were the consumer representatives sufficiently well informed, determined, and persuasive to alter, in a major way, the decisions that would have been taken in their absence. But it would be an error, in fact a serious error, not to recognize that if the future does not belong to the consumer, it will be greatly influenced by his actions and reactions.

There are two ways of tracing the consumer's potential influence, and each is almost certain to have a major impact on the future of health care in the United States—as a user of health care services and as a citizen-voter who will influence legislation, governmental expenditures, and advisory bodies. Years ago, physicians told patients what to do, with no explanations offered and with severe rebukes if their orders were not followed. But the day when the physician was oracle and the patient supplicant is long past. We are now in an early stage of working out appropriate relations between patient and physicians with respect to the responsibilities of individuals to protect their health by living sensibly, to initiate contact with the physician when symptoms appear, and to decide jointly with the physician whether they are willing to undergo certain therapeutic interventions, particularly surgery, when the risks are substantial and the benefits cannot be assured.

The foregoing suggest only a few situations where the consumer has a larger role to play in health care. Additional illustrations involve such matters as calculating the prolongation of life that may necessitate painful interventions, including radical surgery and much-reduced functioning; determining the economic costs that one is willing to incur in order to take advantage of some new, but still unproved, therapy; and estimating trade-offs where medical or surgical intervention might alleviate or even cure certain of one's conditions but at a price that might result in worsening another. In all of these matters and others as well, the physicians of the future must learn, preferably sooner rather than later, that the engagement of the patient is a critical aspect of their practice, and the failure to obtain it will leave them open to criticism, even to malpractice suits. Having been brought up in a tradition that stresses the primacy of the professional, in the area of both knowledge and responsibility, physicians will remain resistant, and there will be nothing easy about the medical profession changing its spots. But it must if the consumer is to be satisfied, and that is always a priority challenge for all who provide services to the public.

A related but distinguishable challenge involves the new and much expanded role of the citizen in the formulation of health policy. Such an expanded role flows directly from the confluence of several trends—the trend to democratization in Western nations; the much enlarged role of government as the source of funds for health care; the previously alluded to increase in the educational level of the citizenry that encourages them to have and voice opinions on matters affecting their own well-being; and the growing skepticism on the part of large segments of the public about whether any interest group— even one held in such high esteem as physicians—can be trusted to act solely for the general, rather than its own, welfare. The question that the United States confronts is not whether the citizenry is going to have a say in the restructuring of the health care system so that it can be made more responsive to its needs and goals, but rather how this more active participation of the citizenry in decisionmaking can be provided in a fashion where the results will, on balance, be constructive.

There are some who believe that the appropriate, even the only, arena for such participation is in the halls of Congress, the arena where national issues are debated and resolved. But many others would insist that state, and even local, governmental bodies are appropriate settings for engaging in such debates and in seeking improved solutions. Admittedly, the government arena is an important setting for the voices of citizens to be heard, for their vote to be cast. But in 1980, approximately 60 percent of the health care industry lies beyond the boundaries of government, in the private and nonprofit sectors. Unless the citizenry were to decide that all power should be transferred to the governmental sphere (as unlikely to happen as it would, in my view, be dysfunctional) greater citizen participation must also be provided in the nongovernmental arena. There, many critical decisions will be made—not once, but continuously—involving consensus about priorities, the allocation of resources, the conditions of access, the distribution of rewards, and the enhancement of quality.

There is no blueprint to show how this objective of greater citizen involvement can be achieved and maintained. What exists are some models of early actions in pursuit of this goal. Some work reasonably well, others are still struggling to find their way. We need not only more experimentation but also a careful monitoring of the results so that the successes can be replicated, the failures not repeated. At this point, one conclusion can be safely ventured. Considerable effort should be made to develop more effective methods of citizen participation in the decisionmaking process involving the health care system, for the citizen-voter has no intention, nor should he, of leaving such matters to be decided solely by physicians and health administrators. Clearly the latter must continue to play major roles, but they can no longer expect society to approve their actions without prior participation.

This review of the bounds within which health policy must be fashioned in the decades ahead contains these clear markings: the importance of avoiding deliberate or inadvertent downgrading of the practice of medicine, which could result in a lower level of professional service; the necessity to develop consensus among critically important groups that will provide the political muscle required for rationalizing the use of resources and assuring the maintenance of quality standards; and experimentation aimed at the constructive involvement of the patient-consumer and citizen-voter, each of whom, if effectively engaged, can contribute a great deal to strengthening the health care system. But beyond these markings, we need to deepen our understanding of the role of services in the economy so that we can point to the positive intervention that promises to contribute to the general welfare by constructive reform of the health care system. The avoidance of error is only the first half of the task that we face.

Reference

Department of Health, Education and Welfare. *Medical Care of Acute Conditions*. (DHEW Pub. no. [PHS] 79-1557, Series 10, no. 129.) Washington, D.C.: Government Printing Office.

HIGH-RISK SCENARIOS FOR THE UNFINISHED AGENDA

Rashi Fein, Ph.D.
Professor of Economics, Harvard Medical School

The fact that health services cannot be stockpiled and held in inventory means that we need a different mode of analysis than that which would apply elsewhere in the economy. Prices, location of producers, access—all are affected in important ways. I recall vividly the difference between the work of two commissions on which I served: One dealing with hunger in America, the other with health care. In the first case, we had a relatively simple task. We could assume that solving the problem did not require that we figure out a way to build grocery stores and get grocers to go to areas where people were hungry. The issue was money or vouchers or food stamps, not distribution networks. In the second case, we did have to concern ourselves with the delivery system, and therefore the activities of that commission required much more time and effort. Dr. Ginzberg explores these matters. His analysis helps us to organize our thinking and to understand the nature of the differences between programs that transfer dollars or provide food stamps and those that offer Medicaid assistance. Future commissions will have an easier task because of his contribution.

Dr. Ginzberg's "prognostication" for the end of the century suggests that he is an incrementalist. He believes that the most likely course—and the wisest course as well—is to expect and seek small changes, small improvements, here and there. Don't misunderstand me: He wants the society to do better and expects that that will occur—but only if we devote energy to improvements at the margin. He feels that if our efforts are focused only on big dreams and major reforms, which he is convinced will not occur, we will miss out on the smaller improvements that are possible. He also believes that if perchance we did succeed in implementing big changes, we would do damage because of the inability to foresee the secondary consequences of new societal interventions. He is a believer in continuity and is leery of discontinuity. I suppose he feels that a quarter of a loaf is better than none, and therefore—and this is important—it is crucial to fight for that quarter. This is an honorable position. Nevertheless, I find it a troublesome one. Dr. Ginzberg gets the incremental progress he favors because of those who call for bigger change. I may not have succeeded in attaining my goals, but I have helped define his position as the middle of the road. It should be clear that I do not use that phrase as a pejorative; the middle of the road is not synonymous with straddling the fence.

None of us can disagree with his cautions. It is dangerous to career down the highway, *and* it is dangerous to drive too slowly. Yet reasonable men and women can differ on the appropriate rate of speed, on the benefits to be achieved from speed, and on the risks we face. The assessment of benefits, of course, depends on one's evaluation of the present state of affairs. Is incrementalism sufficient, or is it an attempt to leap over a chasm in two steps? Is there a chasm, or merely a small depression? John Stuart Mill wrote: "When the object is to raise the permanent condition of a people, small means do not merely produce small effects, they produce no effects at all." Are we not in fact dealing with that kind of issue when we address the medical care sector? We differ on our assessments of the need for change. Perhaps incremental change is all that will occur, but should we not press for more? The answer, of course, is related to the risks we face, and these, in turn, are influenced by conditions internal and external to the health care system. It is the latter, the external conditions, that I focus on.

The prognosis for the year 2000 is essentially an optimistic one. True, it doesn't make me happy. For example, Dr. Ginzberg anticipates relatively little change, by my criteria, in the equity aspect of national health insurance, and I think that achievement of greater equity is a matter of high priority. He also apparently discounts major changes in the social order of which the health sector is a part and which it reflects. Now, I am not a member of the Club of Rome and do not identify with those who prophesy doom. Nevertheless, if not doom, what about gloom?

It is not difficult to project fundamental changes—discontinuities—in our society. Surely the conditions that might lead to such discontinuity do not appear as improbable as they did only a short decade ago. Economists and social observers may feel uncomfortable in mapping the unfamiliar terrain on the other side of the discontinuity, but the contours of that terrain are worth considering. Imagine continuing inflation, or indeed, as a result of actions by OPEC, even more severe inflationary pressures and critical supply shortages. Imagine actions by monetary authorities to control inflation leading to further increases in interest rates. Imagine a severe decline in the housing market; imagine a significant drop in production and an increase in unemployment; imagine the fear that follows upon the heels of a decline in real wealth and savings and an increase in the feeling of powerlessness and uncertainty. Imagine the need to adjust to a shift from growth and expansion to no growth, even decline. It may be unlikely, but it is not outlandish or unthinkable to consider a sharp decline in energy availability as a trigger for this scenario.

None of this requires a fertile imagination. Consider, then, what may follow. It was growth, expansion, the frontier psychology, that enabled this most individualistic nation to develop social programs that helped mitigate inequality. We redistributed in relatively painless fashion out of the fruits of growth and with an air of optimism. We share and believed in upward economic and social mobility, and that very belief helped relieve social and economic tensions and frictions. In a period of stagnation, if not of economic decline, in a period of hunkering down, in a period of pessimism—will we engage in efforts to increase equity? Will social programs wither at the very moment when they become more necessary? What will follow when the have-nots conclude that next year, and in the years to follow, they and their children will remain have-nots? It is certainly not hard to imagine that one consequence will be that each of us tries to hang on to what we have, and we will witness an increasing polarization and militancy and the end of what sense of community still remains.

Thus it is that I conclude that the assumption of continuity, a future like the present, is optimistic. I suggest, however, that the costs of alternative, low-probability but high-risk, scenarios are sufficiently important to warrant their full exploration and consideration. Time in which to make progress on our unfinished agenda may be running out. I would like Dr. Ginzberg to think about how we can best prepare for a social order that may look very different.

THE PHYSICIAN'S CONCERN FOR COSTS
Marvin J. Shapiro, M.D.
Former Chairman, California Blue Shield

Practicing physicians and their organizations have known for a long time that classic economic concepts do not apply to health care. Somewhat naive and lacking in technical know-how in economics, few if any of us have understood why. Certainly, few in medicine grasped that ours was only one rather large part of the economics of services, as contrasted to products.

Physicians have been remarkably unsuccessful in trying to explain to planners, theorists, and legislators why their proposals for improving the health care system were doomed to fail. Dr. Ginzberg has explained why. He points out that societal control in the health care industry has been the responsibility of a combination of government standard-setting and policing by the profession. There can be little dispute that this combination has gradually been losing effectiveness. The public is now inadequately protected in terms of both cost and quality. I would suggest that the time at which the combination began to fail can be placed with some accuracy just fifty years ago, with the birth of Blue Cross and health insurance. At much the same time—and growing even more rapidly—came the technological explosion in medical care. Thus, as the physician had ever less concern about the individual patient's costs, the potential for the physician to initiate expensive care increased dramatically. The resultant astonishing rise in community costs has caused the predictable results and the numerous proposals designed to at least slow the rate of escalation. Dramatic proposals to shift control of the health care industry to the federal government by legislating some form of national health service, or to state governments through rigid controls, or to the marketplace through competition not only have little likelihood of success but carry with them a very high probability of producing chaos and drastic deterioration in quality of care. This leaves us still dependent on government standard-setting and policing by the profession. I agree that government standard-setting has been at least fair and probably needs only modest changes; this means that the work of the profession must be considerably improved. I'm convinced that the needed improvement is possible, and that it has begun.

The American Medical Association, specialty societies, state societies, county societies, and even individual hospital staffs are at present carrying on programs designed to make physicians more aware of costs and to modify physician behavior in such ways as to control costs. These programs are highly commendable and of great value in terms of raising consciousness. However, I submit that in themselves they can have only minimal effect, because in the individual physician-patient relationship other pressures prevail. Because of the pressure from patients and their families to "do everything, doctor, and don't worry about the cost, the insurance will pay for it anyhow," because of the ever-present, frightening specter of malpractice actions, and because of the pressures from the medical-industrial complex to use the elegant, staggeringly expensive new technologies, appropriately or not, in order to amortize their costs and justify their purchase, a very significant part of the approximately $150 billion dollars' worth of health care costs initiated by physicians is initiated against their better judgment in the knowledge that there is no reasonable possibility of benefit to the patient and that in some instances the patient is being exposed to unnecessary risk. Furthermore, there are doctors who are still ordering or performing procedures long since discredited. Since the third parties in general ask nothing more than that there be a physician's order and evidence that the procedure was performed, virtually all these services are being reimbursed. But I believe that some very impressive savings can be achieved by reintroducing into the physician-patient relationship an element that has largely been lost: The physician's concern, and the patient's concern, for the direct cost to the patient. Many others have reached this conclusion and have proposed coinsurance and deductibles as a solution, but I have to agree with Dr. Ginzberg that these have a distinctly limited potential, particularly because of the position of organized labor on first-dollar coverage.

But if the patient and the physician were aware that a contemplated procedure was not likely to be paid for by a third party, and certainly would not be paid except by specific report, in all probability there would be a discussion in depth involving the potential benefit to the patient. The physician would be free of patient pressure arising from the knowledge of insurance payment, and largely free of the pressure from the medical-industrial complex, which depends to a great extent on the existence of insurance. If authoritative professional opinion had previously stated that the procedure was indicated only in special situations, and if it were not applicable to the case being considered, the physician would also largely be relieved of peer pressure and fear of malpractice action. A dramatic decrease in useless services could be anticipated, with great savings and with much-improved quality of care.

With all this in mind, the Professional Affairs Committee of the Blue Shield Association, which had been charged by the Blue Shield board to develop a program directed toward slowing cost escalation, proposed the Medical Necessity Program. The program is based on the fact that most contracts underwriting health care state in one way or another that the contract will cover only medically necessary services, but the committee recognized that virtually no attempt had been made to delineate "medically necessary." Therefore the committee recommended that the most credible and highly respected national professional organizations be requested to review specific procedures and advise the associations if some of the procedures should no longer be paid routinely. The committee decided from the beginning that the Plans should never say "never", but should only change from routine payment to payment by report.

Procedures that might be considered old and discredited, new and unproven, redundant, repetitive, and purely defensive were identified by the committee as deserving evaluation. It decided that the first challenge was to establish the credibility of the approach by considering services still being paid routinely that members of the committee and Plan medical directors felt had become outdated. The American College of

Surgeons, American College of Physicians, American College of Radiology, and American Academy of Family Practice were most cooperative in reviewing and recommending that 28 procedures no longer considered useful should henceforth be paid only by report. It was estimated that if the commerical insurance companies and the government followed the lead, which they have done, the community might be saved some $200 million annually. That figure may be an understatement when one considers that $18 million a year were being paid for just one of the procedures—uterine suspension. The outdated procedures have now been expanded to 107, many of the additions having been first suggested by the societies. The vitally needed cooperation of the specialty societies has continued, and other societies are now participating. The validity of the program seems to have been established.

Now the challenge to the profession and its organizations is to move to the area of the other, much more difficult redundant, repetitive, unproven, and defensive procedures and to determine when a service is of little value because it is inappropriate. It may be possible for some recommendations to be made by individual specialty societies, as before. For some evaluations, ad hoc groups representing several specialties, or representatives of other disciplines may be needed. In some instances members of the general public may also be included, if a decision is one concerning cost effectiveness, morality, and the willingness of the public to expend large amounts of money for relatively little yield in terms of improved health.

Most practicing physicians feel that inhalation therapy is being overused and abused. Intensive care units of all types—beyond question of great value to some patients—may well be overused to the detriment of some patients, and at tremendous cost. The entire large and expanding field of imaging—from old-fashioned x-rays, through radionuclide studies to ultrasound and computerized tomography scanning—might well be studied from the point of view of appropriateness and redundancy. The appropriate work-up of both suspected and diagnosed myocardial infarct could well be scrutinized, to say nothing of improving determinations of when coronary bypass surgery is appropriate, for it, as many of us suspect, there is gross overutilization of services like these, many billions of dollars are involved.

One example might be useful: There is no evidence that establishing a diagnosis of metastatic spread following mastectomy, prior to the development of symptoms, improves the outcome of the patient in any way as compared to instituting palliative therapy after symptoms are apparent. Yet numerous articles in the literature recommend that asymptomatic postmastectomy patients be checked at least once, and in some articles twice, a year for possible metastases, that the checkup include at least a bone scan, and in most of the papers, bone, liver, and lung scans. Some even include brain scan. Annual triple scans of the asymptomatic postmastectomy patients in this country would cost the community at least $200 million, if follow-up was continued for only five years. (The literature leaves the duration of follow-up open). And though there is no evidence that there would be any benefit to any patient, there is evidence that, since scans are less than 100 percent accurate (most series find approximately 20 percent false positives), some asymptomatic women without metastases are given chemotherapy or radiation therapy, with the usual unpleasant side effects—certainly not good-quality care.

Thus for the year 2000 I see societal control of health care still largely a combination of government standard-setting and professional policing, with the work of the profession expanded, improved, and much more effective. Improvement will be due mostly to acceptance by the professionals of a new sense of responsibility to the public for costs and cost effectiveness. There is no doubt that enthusiasts for government control and the marketplace will be with us during the next twenty years, and that from time to time their proposals will surface and be put in place. But most of them will quickly atrophy, perhaps with some residual effects. Professor Ginzberg has given the medical profession and the Blue Shield Plans a real challenge. I think the challenge can and will be met.

2 EQUAL ACCESS TO HEALTH CARE FOR EVERYBODY

Wilbur J. Cohen
Former Secretary U.S. Department of Health,
Education and Welfare

Wilbur J. Cohen, former undersecretary and secretary of the U.S. Department of Health, Education and Welfare, is perhaps best described as the "father of Medicare." Through his efforts and leadership, the Medicare and Medicaid programs moved through Congress to provide affordable health care service to those who needed it most—the elderly and the poor. His career has included service to both government and education, including a lengthy stint with the Social Security Administration. After eight years with the Department of Health, Education and Welfare, Cohen became dean of the University of Michigan School of Education. A member of the executive board of the Institute of Sociological Research, he also has served as cochairman of the Institute of Gerontology at the University of Michigan and Wayne State University. Recipient of numerous awards in health and education, Cohen has authored or coauthored several books and articles, including Retirement Policies in Social Security, Social Security: Programs, Problems and Policies *and* Income and Welfare in the United States.

The idea of comprehensive health insurance—every American protected against the financial consequences of medical costs—began to appear in the United States early in this century. High mortality and morbidity rates, coupled with serious eco-

60

nomic and health problems arising out of urbanization and industrialization, stimulated political action on a wide range of social-reform measures. Mothers' pensions, women's right to vote, abolition of child labor, and workers' accident compensation were major issues. Insurance against the costs of medical care and income loss due to accidents on the job as a substitute for common-law liability developed on a state-by-state basis. It was natural that the health insurance movement followed the state precedent of social insurance with respect to accidents. During the period from 1912 to 1919, several state commissions studied proposals for state health insurance. The American Medical Association briefly flirted with support in 1917 but quickly withdrew its approval. With the "return to normalcy" during the 1920s, the first political opportunity to establish governmental health insurance in the United States on a state basis dissolved.

During the early 1930s, there was widespread belief that it was not actuarially feasible to insure medical costs on a voluntary basis. Despite—or because of—foreign experience, many insurance experts in the private sector were skeptical about, or opposed to, taking the risk of underwriting such insurance coverage. But teachers in Texas, undaunted by the mysteries of actuarial science, approached the solution of the problem on a pragmatic basis and thus led the way to the establishment of Blue Cross and the nationwide acceptance of the insurance principle as applied to medical costs. Neither private health insurance, collective bargaining, or the medical care system of the nation was ever the same again. A new institution had been born that, step-by-step, has precipitated a long and controversial set of policy issues similar in intensity to such other major national issues as federal aid to education, civil rights, abortion, and the equal rights amendment.

The conventional wisdom of the time that any social insurance program would have to be established on a state-by-state basis was unexpectedly overturned by a Supreme Court decision of May 1937 upholding the constitutionality of the taxes and benefits of the old-age insurance system under the Social Security Act. Although the Wagner-Murray Bill of 1939 was predicated primarily upon federally aided state action, this state option died quickly for a second time, and the major new direction for federal action in health insurance superseded the state-by-state approach of the previous forty years.

Not until 1943 was the first significant national health insurance bill introduced into the U.S. Congress, the Wagner-Murray-Dingell Bill. During the period 1943 to 1950, this bill was roundly denounced by the AMA as socialized medicine, compulsion, regimentation, and interference in the doctor-patient relationship. Action on a comprehensive plan was stalemated as a result of AMA opposition, and the idea of a limited health insurance plan covering only the aged was first proposed in 1951. It remained legislatively dormant until 1957 and then rushed into center place in the political campaign of 1960. For four more years it was a key congressional and presidential issue. Then, with the election of Lyndon Johnson in 1964 and the increased number of Democratic congressmen who were elected on his coattails, Medicare became part of American life in 1965.

But the period 1943 to 1965 was nevertheless of key importance in the development of national health policy. The political threat of federal legislative action on health insurance in the mid-1930s and early 1940s, and the economic impact of wage and price controls during World War II (1942–1945) and the Korean War (1950–1952), stimulated private and commercial health insurance plans (Blue Cross, Blue Shield, and commercial carriers) to expand their coverage. Despite the doubts of many private insurance underwriters, employer and union interest in health insurance increased, and health insurance became an accepted institution.

The first presidential message devoted entirely to health was issued in November 1945 by President Harry S. Truman. The message outlined a comprehensive national health program, including national health insurance. During the postwar period, government action occurred at the national level in various health and medical areas (Hill-Burton hospital construction, 1946; public welfare medical assistance, 1950–1965, especially the Kerr-Mills medical assistance bill for the aged, 1960; and disability insurance, 1956). These diverse developments culminated in the enactment by Congress in 1965 of Medicare and Medicaid and in the coverage of physicians under Social Security; the professional standards review organization and health maintenance organization legislation in 1972; and the National Health Planning and Resources Development Act in 1974.

The Medicare legislation of 1965 altered the entire nature of the public-policy discussion about the financing, organization, delivery, and reimbursement of medical services. An ideological Rubicon was crossed in a quantum leap. The event precipitated nationwide acceptance not only of the general idea of comprehensive national health insurance but also, for the first time, of proposals for the basic reorganization of the health care delivery system, changes in the methods of insurance reimbursement for physicians and hospitals, and the support for group practice of medical care through health maintenance organizations (HMOs).

Although the detailed outlines of the acceptable national health insurance plan that is likely to develop in the future still remain shrouded in mystery in 1979, it is probable that public policy in the immediate future will discard two specific approaches. The first is the *exclusive* continued reliance on the private, voluntary insurance mechanism for an adequate handling of *all* responsibilities related to costs, financing, controls, and the availability and effective delivery of care. The second is the *complete* reliance on a public medical *service* approach—such as Great Britain, the Soviet Union, and several other countries employ—in which the costs are financed wholly or largely out of general revenues and the reimbursement of physicians is not on a fee-for-service basis but by salaries.

The provisions of the various health insurance proposals introduced in Congress in recent years not only tend to support this dual-discard contention but also indicate that in the United States some kind of mixed system will very likely evolve, at least initially, utilizing both the public and private sectors. Probably the evolution will proceed on some kind of disjointed incremental basis, with due regard for pragmatic considerations because of the diversity of the economic, political, and social forces at work in connection with the American medical care system. Thus, while the experience of other countries is of vital interest, the United States will most likely diverge in major respects from their patterns.

The allocation of public and private responsibilities in any new and broader national health insurance legislation could take the form incorporated in the Medicare program: Public financing through payroll contributions and general revenues, but with use of private agencies as fiscal intermediaries or payment agencies, not as financial insuring mechanisms. In other words, the federal government would perform the insuring or underwriting function; the private agencies would perform the payment function under conditions specified by Congress in the federal law.

The financing of medical costs will continue to be an issue around which considerable difference of opinion will revolve. Nevertheless, there at least appears to be widespread acceptance that an employer should pay all or a major portion of the costs of health insurance coverage for employees and their families as a form of wage supplement, based on the fact that they can deduct all such costs from taxable income (as a business expense), whereas an individual can deduct only a limited amount. The acceptance of the principle of employer-financed coverage represents a significant change in both public and employer opinion over the past forty years. Employers originally considered that they should finance only a small portion, if any, of the cost of health protection for their employees, and that employees should finance the cost for their dependents; but out of the continuing collective bargaining process this attitude has changed.

Nearly all major proposals for financing a national health insurance plan introduced in the Congress so far would rely on substantial general revenues to assure coverage for low-income persons. It is thus possible, and even probable, that the eventual plan enacted into law will utilize multiple sources of financing, but in what combination remains an open question. Recent interest in the value added tax (VAT) by the chairmen of the House Committee on Ways and Means and the Senate Finance Committee raise new and controversial issues regarding financing of social insurance.

In general, the major national health insurance plans proposed up until now assume that the financing of the plan would come from four sources: (1) employer contributions, (2) employee contributions, (3) federal general revenues, and (4) some state (and possibly local) revenues to pay for services to the medically indigent. This financial design raises two major policy questions:

1. How much of the total costs should be assessed on each of these sources of funds and on what rationale?
2. To what extent, if any, would the employer and employee contributions be collected by nongovernmental agencies or by state and federal public agencies? What implications would arise from these various alternatives?

In 1979, an Advisory Council on Social Security recommended that the costs of Medicare should be financed by an earmarked income tax on individuals and an earmarked corporation income tax, instead of by payroll taxes. Along with proposals to substitute the Social Security taxes by a VAT, it would seem that there will be considerable debate over the methods of financing of Social Security, Medicare, and national health insurance in the near future. Moreover, any decision to change the financing of any program may affect the other two. A great deal may depend on the happenstance of which program comes up for legislative action first and on the contemporary attitude on taxes and expenditures.

In periods of budgetary constraints and high rates of inflation, any proposed national health insurance plan will raise questions about costs, financing, controls, and the quality of medical care that will result in differences of judgment and a need for accommodation of strong conflicting views. Only strong presidential and congressional leadership can resolve these unscientific and political issues in order to achieve enactment of a specific and workable plan.

During the past two years, considerable political and technical efforts have gone into proposals to control rising hospital and other medical costs. Differences have arisen not only between those who favor voluntary as compared to mandatory legislative and administrative controls but also among those who support controls prior to enactment of a national health insurance plan and those who believe such constraints can be achieved only, if at all, through a comprehensive national health insurance program. In any case, the debate over controls and constraints has probably delayed legislative consideration and enactment of any national health insurance plan, while at the same time fanning the flames for further federal action in favor of both comprehensive coverage and catastrophic coverage.

Most people recognize that any comprehensive national health insurance plan will involve some additional expenditures, but there is substantial difference of opinion on both the short-term and long-term cost effects of various proposals. Experience with Blue Cross, Blue Shield, Medicare, Medicaid, and other voluntary and governmental health insurance plans—especially during a period of generally rising prices—has made legislators and others wary of the validity of estimates of future medical care costs, irrespective of the source of the estimates. Many employers and taxpayers fear that costs will rise far more than estimates indicate. There is widespread skepticism as to whether either mandatory or voluntary controls can substantially decrease costs. Many physicians, however, believe that any national health insurance plan may tend to hold down expenditures through control of physicians' fees and hospital reimbursements. And many health professionals say that a much better distribution of services could be achieved within the totals presently being expended if there were changes in the health delivery system. But there is little evidence of rapid fundamental changes. Consequently, it is likely that medical expenditures will rise to beyond 9 percent of the gross national product in the 1980s, and possibly to 10 percent by the year 2000, unless some unforeseen developments occur to restrain inflation in the medical care system.

One of the key issues to be decided by Congress is whether the reimbursement control features of the plan that will be enacted will be supervised by federal personnel *directly* with providers; or as in Medicare, with intermediaries acting as fiscal agents of the federal government; or by allotting funds to the states so that they will have the responsibility of keeping reimbursements and control of costs within bounds; or by giving control directly to the private insurance carriers.

It is not clear at this time which of these approaches to reimbursement control will be favored by consumers, professional associations, congressional policymakers, and federal, state, and local agencies. Of course, it would also be possible to include several variations in the plan and let the choices be made by consumers, states, and providers. There is, however, no concrete evidence which of these approaches will produce the most effective cost controls.

The differences of opinion over the cost of any national health insurance plan focus largely on the impact of its particular provisions on the elasticity of demand for medical services, the methods for reimbursing providers, and the effectiveness of cost controls. Any plan that provides medical services to people not now receiving them is reasonably certain to increase costs. Critics of the public-sector approach usually claim that any plan that relies solely or substantially on full, or nearly full, insurance of costs under governmental responsibility will weaken personal responsibility for conservative financial administration, and hence, that any comprehensive national health insurance plan will increase costs.

On the other hand, there are those who believe that a national health insurance plan could be drawn up with appropriate provisions to constrain cost increases. These people argue for limitations on fees, restraints on hospital utilization, budgeting of institutional costs, salary or per capita payments instead of fees, group practice plans instead of solo practice, and other changes in the delivery of services. But irrespective of what various groups think *should be* done to change the health delivery system, it would be prudent to plan for some initial increase in expenditures under *any* national health insurance plan that may be enacted. By phasing in the scope and coverage of services offered in a comprehensive plan, it might be feasible to keep the net annual increases within politically acceptable bounds over a number of years.

The formulation and administration of a national health insurance plan raises a host of complex issues, some of which are so personal or so diffuse that it is not possible to isolate all the forces and factors involved. Health care is not a commodity but a sensitive service; many would say it is the most significant service rendered by one individual for another. It is difficult to compare it in importance with any other service, and the health professional, patient, economist, taxpayer, and legislator will evaluate it differently, diverge on innumerable aspects of the health insurance issue, and disagree strongly on key matters of national health policy.

Despite numerous variations, each of the many major national health insurance plans that have been proposed or considered over the past forty-five years can be classified under one or another of the following general models:

1. Employs federal tax credits, federal subsidies, or vouchers to encourage universal acceptance of coverage on a voluntary basis.
2. Allows individuals and employers to be covered voluntarily under a broadened Medicare plan along the lines of Medicare Part B.
3. Mandates employers to cover employees and their families under private plans, with federal general revenues covering the remainder of the population.
4. Extends Medicare to cover employees and the self-employed under the Social Security system for major-medical (catastrophic) insurance coverage and to provide a federally financed system of medical care coverage for low-income persons, with the residual coverage handled through the voluntary system.
5. Utilizes the Social Security system to collect contributions from employers and employees and to pay benefits, with federal general revenues covering the remainder of the population.
6. Broadens the coverage of Medicare on a population-age basis by lowering the age requirement or extending coverage to mothers and children and other age groups.
7. Utilizes federal tax or subsidy arrangements to induce each state to provide health insurance coverage to its citizens, with a variety of options to states and individuals.

In any of these plans, the following payment and reimbursement features can be incorporated separately or in some combination:

1. Private plans (Blue Cross, Blue Shield, and commercial carriers) could be used as fiscal intermediaries for the federal or state government to provide for the payment of benefits on a managerial fee basis.
2. State agencies could serve as insurance carriers or fiscal intermediaries.
3. Health maintenance organizations (HMOs) could be chosen by the employer or employee, or through collective bargaining, as the service unit for providing care to enrolled persons.
4. Reimbursement of physicians could be accomplished through a variety of methods, such as fee-for-service, capitation, salary, hours of service, or some combination of these methods.
5. One or more state health insurance plans, or HMOs, could be established as benchmarks or standards for comparison with other plans.

These are, of course, simplified expressions of often highly complicated technical proposals. They are, however, the elements that can make the plan work effectively and acceptably. They deserve more careful consideration by advocates and opponents.

Proposals for national health insurance invariably generate a wide range of extended and critical remarks on the volatile issue of the respective advantages and disadvantages of public and private responsibilities. The issue has been persistent and controversial in many questions of social policy throughout American history, but it is fair to say that on the question of national health insurance, the debate over public versus private obligations has raised special emotional and ideological arguments.

Although political and ideological factors are frequently discussed in general terms relating to power, authority, and responsibility, many other issues come into play in discussions of national health insurance, such as pluralism, centralization versus decentralization, cost implications, managerial effectiveness and economy, administrative costs and paperwork, and adaptability to local circumstances and attitudes.

The basic view of the American Medical Association concerning national health insurance may be simply stated as being antigovernmental: That is, the AMA favors as little governmental participation in the program as is feasible. Most physicians—as independent, business-oriented, self-employed professionals—have strongly indicated their belief in the general philosophic contention that "that government is best which governs least." They also firmly believe, as do many people in other fields, that government is generally more wasteful, inefficient, and expensive than private enterprise. Moreover, they claim that the regulatory function exercised by government fosters rules that are rigid and inappropriate in relation to the varying and special circumstances of medical practice. The views of the AMA are generally shared by insurance companies, pharmaceutical-manufacturing companies, and, to a large extent, by proprietary hospitals and nursing homes. Although these opinions may not be supported by incontrovertible facts pertinent to medical care, they are strongly held and have emotional and ideological shadings that appear in the election literature of political campaigns. They are repeated often and become widely accepted as the conventional wisdom, not requiring documentation.

The proponents of public-sector responsibility in a national health insurance plan believe, on the other hand, that only through the public sector can equity to all participating individuals be assured. Equity in this context means assurance of similar treatment of individuals in similar circumstances with respect to financing, access to the delivery system, quality of care, adjudication of grievances, and similar matters. Private plans cannot meet this objective of equity.

To simplify the issue, we can say that there is a significant difference in approach and in values between those who emphasize *efficiency* and those who emphasize *equity* in the implementation of a national health insurance plan. Neither group would exclude outright the consideration of the other's values, but there is an important difference in the weight each group gives to the concepts of efficiency and equity.

Recourse to history, an examination of foreign experience and domestic programs, reference to human nature—and the implications these have for the future—all are open to various interpretations and make objective evaluation of these two concepts imprecise. Moreover, since personal values are so much a part of this assessment, it is difficult to avoid emotionalism—efficiency and equity mean different things to different people. Neither concept, however, is pushed by its adherents to an ultimate conclusion: There appear to be limitations or exceptions to each concept that the adherents make regarding the given elements in a proposal.

Here are two of innumerable illustrations: Those who strongly argue for a particular national health insurance proposal that will cost less because it will be handled by nongovernmental agencies do not move to the logical conclusion of advocating a single agency to collect premiums and thereby save millions of dollars in administrative costs. Nor do those who believe that a governmental plan should insure equitable treatment of patients or contributors necessarily go further and apply the concept of equity to the providers of care. Which is more equitable, uniform payments, or differential payments to providers in different geographical areas? Cost and historical developments also play a significant role in evaluating the importance of equity and efficiency.

My own experiences in implementing health, education, and welfare programs, especially during the 1960s, have led me to the strong conviction that efforts to put into effect a large-scale program on a single day can lead to major administrative difficulties and extensive disappointment. There are errors of judgment; personnel and facilities do not work out as intended; unforeseen delays occur; costs rise; and unforeseen local, state, and special problems develop that require time and infinite patience for solution. It is therefore more effective to plan for a realistic, step-by-step implementation in the law that takes into account the realities of human limitations.

The incremental evolution of future American health and medical care coverage seems less clear, in view of the many possible ways of handling key policy and management problems. One incremental step that has been suggested is the initial coverage of catastrophic medical care costs along the lines of major-medical insurance coverage (proposed by Louisiana's Senator Russell Long and Connecticut's Senator Abraham Ribicoff); another is the comprehensive coverage of all maternity costs and the coverage of children up to the ages of six, twelve, or eighteen (proposed by Congressman James Scheuer and Senator Jacob Javits of New York, and others). These two elements could be joined into various combinations of coverages and costs, including reduction of the eligibility age for Medicare coverage from sixty-five to sixty-two or sixty. The major point, however, is that there are various means of arriving at comprehensive coverage over a period of time.

Supporters of a comprehensive national health insurance plan have vigorously opposed enactment of a catastrophic coverage plan as a single step to accompany Medicare, claiming that such a federal plan would exacerbate rising costs by emphasizing institutional and high-cost services and would delay enactment of comprehensive coverage. Nevertheless, catastrophic coverage has wide acceptance in congressional circles. It would not be impossible to conceive of a publicly administered catastrophic coverage plan financed as part of Medicare, along with a comprehensive mandated employer plan for basic hospital and medical services. Another type of plan, which has not been given any attention, is a state-by-state plan, obtained by a federal credit offset tax to assure that all states would enact state unemployment insurance plans. There are other possible combinations and adaptations of federal-state and public-private sector plans that may surface under pressures for political compromises among the different parties in the political vortex.

Despite the delays and controversy, the establishment of some kind of comprehensive national health insurance plan still seems to me to be inevitable. The questions are when and how.

The eventual plan I prefer would cover everyone in the nation from birth to death: the rich and the poor, the young and the old, the middle-income earner and the middle-aged, all minorities, everyone living in urban, suburban, and rural areas, whether working at home, in large corporations, small businesses, domestic service, or migratory labor. The coverage should be universal and should eliminate costly eligibility determinations and delay in providing services.

A national health insurance plan that I believe is both responsible and responsive would be based upon the following general principles:

1. *Breaking the barrier between paying for health care and being eligible for service.* One of the key purposes of a national health plan is, as far as possible, to arrange the prepayment of health costs when an individual is working so that basic financial considerations would not be a major problem during illness and no complicated procedures would be necessary for the unemployed or nonemployed.

2. *Requiring the employee and the self-employed to pay part of the costs.* This would assure the individual of a statutory and political right to benefits without a means test. By having large numbers of people pay small amounts over a long period of time, all individuals could be assured of coverage for comprehensive medical care protection. Such a plan would, as Sir Winston Churchill said, "bring the magic of the averages to the rescue of the millions."

3. *Requiring the employer to pay a reasonable part of the costs.* The employer's contributions would still be deductible from federal and state taxes as a business expense. The employer should be involved in the financing and planning of community health services and be concerned about adequate access to health services for his employees and their families and for health services at the employing unit.

4. *Requiring the general public to contribute a significant part of the cost.* Contributions from federal general revenue, or an earmarked income tax, would guarantee that individuals with no or little income would receive equal access to health services on the same basis as those with more adequate income. The stigma of poverty and welfare would thus be removed from the medical care system. Medicaid in its present form could at the same time be substantially reduced and eventually eliminated.

5. *Requiring that employee and employer contributions to the plan be handled as separate, identifiable additions to Social Security contributions.* This would greatly reduce the

cost of collecting contributions, which now takes place through hundreds of separate arrangements administered by private insurance agencies—an unnecessary, costly, inefficient, and wasteful procedure. A single federal system of collecting contributions through Social Security would be more economical than the present patchwork system, and it could reduce the administrative costs of universal coverage by over $1 billion a year.

6. *Providing for universal coverage and eligibility to services by federal law solely and simply by virtue of legal residence in the United States.* Universal coverage would simplify the eligibility process, reduce accounting, and keep administrative costs to a minimum. One eligibility card and one reimbursement form for physicians and other providers would be both feasible and desirable. No individual would lose eligibility because of any change in employment or because of unemployment or nonemployment.

7. *Assuring that access to service for all persons throughout the nation would be determined by universal rules.* Uniform, nationwide contributions to the health security system should be accompanied by uniform, nationwide standards of access to services. Interpretation of these standards could be delegated to state, local, or federal health agency personnel; but an individual would be assured of a fair hearing before a federal agency on matters in dispute and of an appeal for judicial review by federal courts on matters of law. Due process and equal treatment would be guaranteed to everyone, irrespective of color, age, sex, education, or background.

8. *Providing for a broad range of medical services, with specific arrangements for extending services over a reasonable period of time.* Although comprehensive medical service is a desirable objective, the immediate attainment of that goal as part of eligibility under a national health program is simply not feasible. Any national health program should therefore include specific provisions for a step-by-step expansion of services such as out-of-hospital prescription drugs, nursing-home care, dental care, and other similar services that require planning and organi-

zation for their universal availability. Such planning must, of course, be coordinated with projects for training health personnel, building appropriate facilities, recruiting and redeploying personnel, and developing health maintenance organizations.

9. *Providing for innovative, economical, and efficient methods of organizing and delivering medical care.* Financial incentives should be provided for the expansion of ambulatory and outpatient care, improved emergency services, health maintenance organizations, salary and capitation payments, multiphasic screening, periodic examinations, and community-sponsored, coordinated plans for health education, family planning, nutrition, and environmental concerns. Nurses and other health personnel should be encouraged to provide more effective leadership in community health education programs.

10. *Encouraging and accelerating plans to increase personnel in the health fields.* Financial incentives should be made available for the enlargement of training facilities in order to produce more physicians, nurses, dentists, and other health personnel, including physicians' assistants, aides, technicians, and allied health workers. Particular attention should be given to training more members of minorities and women for employment in the health fields and for other opportunities to participate in the health care system. Medical, nursing, and other schools that train health personnel must establish career incentives and program arrangements to assist in the more rational distribution of personnel and services.

11. *Providing opportunities for the consumer, as taxpaper and patient, to play a significant role in policy formulation and administration of the health system.* Health care is too important a service to be the sole province of any one professional or bureaucratic group, no matter how well trained or well intentioned that group may be. Many questions relating to health care are of critical concern to the consumer: How effectively is the money contributed to health service being spent? Is the administration of health care efficient? Is the consumer assured dignity and privacy by those who provide the care? How are priorities

determined? And there are a host of other questions relating to the diagnosis and treatment of disease or disability. A more effective partnership among the professional, the consumer, and the bureaucrat must be developed so that the public can receive the quality of medical care it needs and deserves.

12. *Assuring health personnel reasonable compensation and opportunities for professional practice, advancement, and the exercise of humanitarian and social responsibility.* The components in a national health program should be designed to provide the highest quality of medical care, with both individuals and groups using initiative, working for professional advancement, and dispensing health care with a creative sense of social responsibility. Those who provide services should receive fair and reasonable compensation in relation to their ability, responsibility, and productivity. They should be able to choose the method of their remuneration. The rate and method of their compensation should be adjusted periodically in relation to changes in program costs, the cost of living, and their own productivity. Various incentives should be provided those who offer medical care to encourage the establishment of such groups as health maintenance organizations.

13. *Encouraging effective professional participation in the formulation of guidelines, standards, rules, regulations, forms, procedures, and organization.* There should be widespread participation by all health personnel in the formulation of policy at the highest levels and at every rank of administration. A sense of cooperative participation among personnel should be fostered to overcome hierarchical considerations and invidious distinctions based on income, education, or prestige. The nursing profession, as a prime example, should be encouraged to assume a stronger leadership role in relating health services to individual family and community needs.

14. *Requiring state and area health agencies to take affirmative leadership in providing for effective delivery of medical services.* A nationwide health insurance plan *cum* health care system should utilize state and area health

agencies to stimulate the availability and coordination of services, set standards for personnel and services, and handle complaints, grievances, and other local problems.

15. *Fostering a pluralistic and flexible system of administration.* Widely divergent ideas about how medical care can best be administered exist in various parts of the United States, among health care personnel generally and among the public at large. We should not seize any one method or system as the best for everyone or for all time. As science and technology continue to develop new methods of diagnosis and treatment, new drugs, and new systems of delivery, we should be willing and able to adapt our arrangements to respond to shifting needs and styles.

A national health insurance plan is not the panacea to solve all the problems of medical care in the United States. The continuing increase in demand for medical services drawn from a short-run, inelastic supply will continue to create rising price and cost pressures into the foreseeable future. Changes in organization, delivery, and access to services to meet the changing demand will not occur overnight. We must develop a long-range plan.

Health education and preventive health care must meanwhile be expanded so that the available medical personnel and facilities will be able to handle acute and chronic sickness and disability. We must also make an effective effort to distribute medical services in a manner that is more rational and socially conscious than the way it is being done at present. Through a national health plan we could focus our planning and our priorities for a more intelligent and equitable distribution of the miracles of medical science to the American people.

Benefits under national health insurance should be phased into operation by a predetermined schedule in the law, which takes into account the progress made under existing federal health legislation. Important new benefits should begin preferably between April and October, and preferably on July 1, in order to avoid the initial impact of the high volume of claims and payment during the high-morbidity period of November to March.

The federal administrative authority for the program should be invested in a board of three to five persons, rather than in a single administrator, to avoid the implications of rule by a "czar of medicine." The federal board should be in operation a number of months before any major new benefits or policies are put into effect.

A health insurance benefits advisory council should make a report each year with any recommendations on the operation of the plan. Every five years, an independent advisory council should review the program and report its recommendations to the President and the Congress. The membership of the council should follow that provided by law for the Advisory Council on Social Security.

Any national health insurance plan utilizing earmarked contributions should not be subject to short-range budgetary considerations merely to decrease or increase overall governmental budget deficits or surpluses.

A separate health appropriations bill should be processed by the Congress to ensure that all health legislation is considered in relation to every aspect of health and medical care. This would mean, for example, including the medical budgets for the Defense Department and the Veterans Administration in this overall consideration.

The national health insurance bill eventually to be enacted by Congress has not yet been introduced or drafted. Judging by past experience, the Congress is likely to include some important and unforeseen elements in any final piece of legislation that takes into account the forces of influence and compromise that affect the legislative and political process. Administrators of the eventual plan must be ready to implement the unexpected.

THE GOALS NOW: HEALTH STATUS AND QUALITY OF LIFE

Julius B. Richmond, M.D.
Assistant Secretary for Health and Surgeon General,
U.S. Department of Health and Human Services

The real goal of a national health insurance plan is to improve health status and the quality of life by assuring people access to care. The programs of the 1960s had some problems, as large new programs always will, but before Medicare and Medicaid, there were wide disparities in the use of services. Today, if we look at utilization of services among the poor and the elderly, there is far more equity in access to physicians' services and hospitals across income groups than before, and although direct medical services cannot take all the credit for improved health status, we must be doing something right.

We have just issued a Surgeon General's report, *Healthy People.* It starts with the sentence: "The health of the American people has never been better."

- Life expectancy is rising and our elderly are growing older.
- The infant mortality rate continues to drop; it is now 13.6 per 1,000 live births. The rate is clearly related to the availability and use of prenatal care and infant care, which has been made available to large numbers of low-income women through Medicaid. The number of poor women who begin their care in the first trimester of pregnancy is steadily rising.
- Deaths from cardiovascular disorders have declined by 22 percent during the past decade.

Many of the key policymakers during the Medicare-Medicaid debates knew that a financing program alone would not assure that services would be available to people who needed them. The 1960s saw a series of innovative programs designed to develop service delivery capability for low-income people and people who lived in underserved areas. We had what I call a bumper crop of health legislation. These programs included the community mental health and retardation legislation, neighborhood health centers—now the highly successful community health centers program, the health programs connected with Head Start, children and youth centers, the high-risk maternity programs, the regional medical programs, and comprehensive health planning. Small wonder that we are still having some indigestion from attempting to absorb all this, and even more that followed.

Public policymakers also recognized the need to make provision for an adequate supply of health professionals, and in anticipation of the financing programs, the federal government in 1963 began its support of health manpower legislation, which during the sixties spurred the development of new health professions like that of the nurse practitioner. Again we did remarkably well; we now have largely overcome the shortages of health personnel, and some are apprehensive about an oversupply.

Most important historically is the change in attitudes of providers, consumers, and government. There is now a consensus, which did not exist in the early 1960s, that we can't just talk insurance or financing. Any national health plan, whether financed publicly, privately, or in combination, must address, or be accompanied by, programs that ensure that services are available. It must also improve the efficiency and effectiveness of delivery, determine that resources are used rationally, devise means to incorporate properly new and rapidly developing health technologies, enhance quality, and stress community and individual health prevention and promotion.

Providers—particularly physicians—although they initially opposed Medicare, have indeed cooperated. There are problems with physician participation in Medicaid, but almost all physicians participate in Medicare. Professional standards review organizations could not work without their support, and the majority of physicians now accept the need for some type of national health plan. In addition, they have been widely supportive of government health prevention and promotion programs: immunizations, maternity and child health programs, and others. The historical resistance of professional groups to governmental interventions has been emphasized, but nevertheless we don't hear any groundswell for the repeal of Medicare and Medicaid.

Consumers have also developed new attitudes. No longer is the consumer the silent voice, the receiver of care rather than the participant. Interest in personal health habits and occupational safety, as well as active involvement in health planning and in various federal, state, and local advisory boards are clear indications of these trends.

If I look back to the time when I was in medical school in the 1930s, when the armamentarium of the physicians was very limited, and compare that period with today, not only has medical technology been revolutionized, but the entire structure of health services delivery and financing has changed. In those days infectious and communicable disease took a heavy toll of children, and life expectancy was about sixty, contrasted with today's seventy-three. Hospitals were institutions for the dying and only beginning to effect cures. The physician-to-population ratio was lower than it had been in the first decade of the century. Except for the school teachers in Dallas, few had any form of health insurance, and many families were frequently wiped out by medical care costs. Most health workers earned substandard wages and had to depend on public aid to survive. One of the best summaries of that era is the report of the Committee on the Costs of Medical Care in 1932, which laid the groundwork for many of the programs that were implemented in the 1960s.

If we plan wisely and use our resources carefully, we will not only have a national health insurance program, but one that will address *health status* as well as *financial access to care*.

CURRENT CHANGES IN THE SYSTEM
Edward J. Connors
President, Sisters of Mercy Health Corporation

The historical developments from the 1930s to the mid-1960s as related by Secretary Cohen carry important lessons for those now in the field who tend to take health insurance for granted or do not have the advantage of having experienced the growth and improvement in health insurance that was accomplished through private initiative, concern, and commitment. I do not agree with the analysis that "the political trend of federal legislative action" deserves the credit ascribed to it here.

The relationship between "fundamental changes in the health delivery system" and national health insurance has not been adequately addressed. It is possible that more fundamental changes are already under way or have already occurred than has been suggested. For example, a fundamental restructuring of hospital ownership, governance, and management has been in progress now for several years. Multiunit systems currently control at least 40 per cent of all the beds in acute nongovernmental hospitals in the United States, and the trend is just beginning. Control of meaningful capital expenditures on the part of hospitals is already a reality, partly through the Health Systems Agencies created by the National Health Planning and Resources Development Act, but also as the result of voluntary action by multiunit systems, effective voluntary interinstitutional cooperation, and support of planning restrictions by private third-party payers.

Alternative delivery systems, particularly health maintenance organizations, are also multiplying at an accelerated rate. Despite unnecessary and unwarranted requirements included in legislation that was presumably intended to encourage the initiation and growth of HMOs, this movement is receiving the active support of major industry, thoughtful hospitals, and some physician groups. It seems likely that the number of competitive alternatives will double or triple with respect to the percentage of the population covered during the 1980s, if they are allowed to develop as a constructive response by providers of health care.

In addition, more-appropriate utilization of facilities and services is being significantly addressed by Blue Cross and Blue Shield Plans, Medicare and Medicaid, and by the emerging professional standards review organizations. Appropriate utilization is at the crux of cost containment, and current efforts, albeit imperfect, may represent the most significant and promising attempts to influence utilization of facilities and services that have been undertaken in any health system in the world.

Moreover, the quality of institutionalized care is an accepted mandate of responsible hospital boards of trustees. Coupled with outside standards promulgated by such voluntary agencies as the Joint Commission on the Accreditation of Hospitals, the commitment to quality by governing boards stands in my opinion as an extraordinary contribution to the public interest.

The principles outlined by Secretary Cohen to guide the establishment of a comprehensive national health insurance plan for the future may well be in conflict with one another. For example, providing for innovative, economical, and efficient methods of organizing and delivering medical care calls for a level of flexibility and risk taking that cannot be found, to my knowledge, in any system that has nationalized the financing of health care services. Also, although "fostering a pluralistic and flexible system of administration" appears to be a highly desirable and laudable principle, experience would seem to indicate that its achievement is very unlikely in the presence of certain other principles enumerated by Secretary Cohen, particularly "nationwide rules to assure access to service" and the requirement that the general public should contribute a significant portion of the cost through taxes. These potential conflicts of principles should be examined in detail in the public debate of any proposals for national health insurance entitlements.

II PUBLIC HEALTH

3 EXPLICIT GOALS FOR PREVENTION AND PUBLIC HEALTH

Donald A. Henderson, M.D., M.P.H.
Dean, Johns Hopkins School of Hygiene and
Public Health

Dr. Donald A. Henderson headed the World Health Organization's global smallpox eradication campaign for a decade before assuming the post of dean of the Johns Hopkins University School of Hygiene and Public Health in 1977. As chief health officer of the WHO program, he planned and carried out one of the most ambitious undertakings in medical history—freeing the world from smallpox. During his first year in directing the WHO campaign, an estimated 10 to 15 million smallpox cases occurred throughout the world, with at least 2 million persons dying from the disease in more than forty countries in Latin America, Africa, and Asia. The disease now is all but medical history. The last case of the killing, blinding, more serious form of smallpox, known as variola major, occurred in October 1975 in Bangladesh. Although cases of variola minor, the less serious strain, persisted in Ethiopia and Somalia through October 1977, certification of the eradication of this strain, following two years of surveillance and research, was announced late in 1979. Dr. Henderson also served with the U.S. Department of Health, Education and Welfare's Center for Disease Control, serving as chief of the epidemic intelligence service, and then as chief of the surveillance section. In these capacities, he was actively involved in efforts to combat Asian influenza, infectious and serum hepatitis, and measles, as well as in the conquest of poliomyelitis.

87

On October 26, 1979, director-general Halfdan Mahler of the World Health Organization (WHO) announced from Nairobi, Kenya: "I am confident in stating that as of today, smallpox has been eradicated throughout the world—that for the first time in history, a disease has been eradicated from the earth. So far as is known, the only remaining smallpox virus is now confined in glass vials in seven laboratories under conditions of high security." The deliberate elimination of a disease, notably one so devastating as this, is a unique event in medical history—the ultimate triumph of preventive medicine. Credit for this achievement properly belongs to a public health team of field staff, scientists, and administrators of the World Health Organization and of countries on every continent.

The achievement of smallpox eradication has given a new impetus to the World Health Organization and to countries throughout the developing world to undertake more aggressive and far-reaching programs in disease prevention. A direct outgrowth is the Expanded Program on Immunization. Its goal for a decade hence is annual vaccination of 90 percent of the world's 100 million newborns against six diseases—diphtheria, pertussis, tetanus, measles, poliomyelitis, and tuberculosis. Meanwhile, a promising cooperative global program of research has begun, coordinated by WHO, to discover improved methods for prevention and treatment of the principal tropical parasitic diseases, leprosy and diarrhea. These programs, as well as other efforts, give priority to prevention and, as a less favored alternative, inexpensive therapies, self-administered or dispensed by health auxiliaries. For countries with limited resources, recognition has come, too often belatedly, that their delivery of health services cannot be patterned after those of the industrialized world. A health service based on hospitals and curative medicine, offering even modest levels of service, requires enormous resources. Illustrative is the experience of one African country that was provided a magnificent 500-bed hospital for its capital city. It was opened with fanfare and fulsome expressions of gratitude to the donor country. Today it sits empty. To operate the hospital to serve a comparative handful of patients—less than 1 percent of the population—required virtually all the country's trained health manpower and one-half of its total budget for health.

The industrialized countries have not been faced with the same stark options that confront the developing world. Money and manpower have been plentiful, and steadily increasing resources could be allocated for the development of progressively more sophisticated curative services. Billions have been expended for the construction of hospitals, in the development of drugs and diagnostic devices, in the training of clinicians and support staff. The past decade has witnessed the development of countless brilliant new interventions in curative medicine—organ transplantation, cancer chemotherapy, intensive care units, computerized axial tomography (CAT) scanners, and renal dialysis, to note but a few. More are on the drawing boards. The faltering human machine is now serviced by a magnificently skilled and equipped industry prepared to effect miracles in repair and restoration. An increasing constituency argues, however, that all defective human machines should have partial, if not full, access to this industry without experiencing bankruptcy. The necessity of some system of national health insurance to provide some degree of universal coverage is acknowledged to be both a societal and political priority.

That we do not now have such a plan recognizes, in part, the harsh reality of Powell's law, a law that is implicitly appreciated but seldom bluntly expressed. Enoch Powell's law states simply that the demand for "free" (i.e., insurance-paid or tax-paid) health care is infinite and can never be met. Or, as stated another way by a recent British Royal Commission: "Whatever the expenditure on health care, demand is likely to rise to meet and exceed it. To believe that one can satisfy the demand for health care is illusory ..." The bitter realization of finite resources and infinite demand is a fact with which we have only tentatively begun to grapple. And the hour is late.

For the developing world, the problems are comparable but the options more obvious. Perhaps from them there is a greater truth to be learned. Their only possible course of action is to direct their energies toward prevention and the application of inexpensive therapies, inexpensively dispensed. Ought there to be a similar redirection of our own future strategy—toward increasing substantially the resources we allocate for manpower development, research, and program implementation in favor of those activities that will keep the human machines out of costly repair shops or, at least, will minimize the use of these repair shops? Certainly neither this nor any other strategy will negate Powell's law. But have we any real choice but to make a far more substantial, deliberate investment in disease prevention and health promotion if we are even to begin to meet rising expectations? Progress through disease prevention and health promotion is less visible, less newsworthy than the drama associated with a heart transplant or the reattachment of a severed limb. To develop and sustain support for successful measures in prevention requires vision, intelligence, imagination, and maturity.

Paradoxically, the saga of smallpox eradication may itself have been unfortunate in encouraging among some the belief that somewhere, sometime, "magic bullets"—vaccines, drugs, procedures—can be found or applied that will dramatically eliminate the naturally occurring insults to the human machine. It is evident that there are only a few disease problems in this country for which one can anticipate such breakthroughs. And global eradication of any other disease, in my opinion, is out of the question in the twentieth century. I propose that it would be constructive if we eradicated the beguiling word "eradication" and focused our energies on the development of necessarily multifaceted, long-term programs for disease prevention and control.

I believe that if we are to make real progress in programs of disease prevention, we badly need specific objectives, clearly stated, and specified time frames for achievement. We then can assess how well or how poorly the programs are functioning and adapt and modify them accordingly. During the past decades in which curative medicine has been dominant, we have identified few such goals. This is not surprising, for practically and philosophically, preventive medicine and curative medicine function differently. Curative medicine has as its clients sick patients who present themselves seeking repair. Success is basically measured in terms of the proportion who are improved or cured—measurements that are comparatively simple. Preventive medicine, however, is concerned with a total population, among whom some seek better health but most are passive or indifferent until they become ill. Success in prevention must be measured in terms of a reduction in the numbers within a total population who die or become sick or disabled. To measure the degree of success of programs and determine which of several possible factors may have been responsible is far more difficult than it is in curative medicine. Because interest and concern for programs in prevention have been vestigial at best, efforts to establish goals and to assess progress have likewise been vestigial. Symptomatic of this is the formulation of objectives in terms of meaningless slogans rather than practicable objectives that might serve to guide the direction and management of the programs. A classic example is the World Health Organization's recent, pretentious "Health for All by the Year 2000."

The goals, to be useful, must be clear in identifying achievement, not simply activity. For the smallpox program, the goal was "0" cases, not the performance of "X" number of vaccinations, but health officials and the press alike had surprising difficulty in accepting this—a report that so many million people had been vaccinated was more impressive, more tangible. This phenomenon is not unique to the international scene. The U.S. Childhood Immunization Program until just a few years ago focused almost exclusively on the millions who were being vaccinated, almost to the point of ignoring whether or not there were fewer cases of disease. Once it was clear to all that the ultimate objective was a reduction in cases of disease, the focus of activity changed. Investigations began to determine the cause of the program's failures—that is, the cases that were still occurring. Were they concentrated in one age group? In a section of a state or county? Among a particular economic group? Were they individuals who had failed to be vaccinated, or could it be that the vaccine was of diminished efficacy? In the smallpox eradication campaign, when we sought answers for each of these questions, it quickly became apparent that program strategy required change. The answers differed from country to country and within different parts of the same country. Accordingly, the programs themselves were continually modified so that as time went on, national programs assumed quite different forms and, even within a given country, the programs varied in character from area to area.

Guidance of program planning and management by means of a surveillance system that monitors disease incidence would seem to be essentials of any program. And yet, as recently as 1967, we determined that not more than 1 percent of all small-pox cases were being reported—that we had that year, not 131,000 cases but some 10 to 15 million cases. Data about vaccinations performed that year were far more complete. To develop an effective and useful disease surveillance system took years and considerable work. In the end, it proved to be the key to success in the program.

National goals in prevention, stated in terms of reasonable expectations and a reasonable time frame, have been nonexistent. Assessment of progress and measurement of achievement have been all but ignored. It is assumed, for example, that our costly, far-flung nutrition programs must be conferring benefit. After all, calories, vitamins, and minerals are being ingested by the needy in great quantities through the medium of school lunch programs, food stamp programs, "Meals on Wheels," and many others. All this must be doing good. But data to support this assumption are sparse. Studies that compare programs as to relative cost and effectiveness are lacking. Lest we assume that the benefits are intrinsically too obvious to warrant the need for monitoring effectiveness and cost, we need only refer to the experience we have had with routine physical examinations. These were, and in some quarters still are, lauded as the cornerstone of a comprehensive program in prevention. Yet only recently, a study in England was reported in which two comparable groups were evaluated as to health status—one group that had had comprehensive routine physical examinations and a second group that had not. The investigators, over time, were unable to identify any difference in the health status of the two.

So long as we persist in vaguely defined, ill-assessed preventive enthusiasms that, uncritically, appear to be the right thing to do, comparatively little will be achieved at great expense.

I welcome the July, 1979, *Surgeon General's Report on Health Promotion and Disease Prevention* for its courage in setting specific, quantitative, measurable goals to be achieved within a defined period of time. Undoubtedly these will be debated as to relevance and magnitude by different interested groups, but they do represent a definitive point of departure.

More needs to be done in setting explicit subgoals that can be used to monitor and guide specific interventions. Even as they stand, each of the stated goals implies action and a measurable end point, and they make a stark contrast with targets such as WHO's stated mission of assuring "the complete physical, social, and mental well-being of all peoples."

The surgeon general's report states goals in terms of reduced mortality and disability rates to be achieved by 1990. They are defined for each of five age groups:

1. Infants—To reduce infant mortality by at least 35 percent, to fewer than 9 per 1,000 live births
2. Children 1 to 14 years old—To reduce deaths by at least 20 percent, to fewer than 34 per 100,000
3. Adolescents and young adults—To reduce deaths among people ages fifteen to twenty-four by at least 20 percent
4. Adults—To reduce deaths among people twenty-five to sixty-four by at least 25 percent
5. Old adults—To reduce the average annual number of days of restricted activity due to acute and chronic conditions by 20 percent, to fewer than thirty days per year for people aged sixty-five and older

The overall objectives represent readily measurable death and disability indicators, but each is prefaced in terms of improvement of health so that, ultimately, rates of death and disability will be lowered. Here, for the first time, are federally proposed national benchmarks by which state and local progress can be continually monitored, problem areas identified, and resources more rationally allocated.

The report expands at length on preventable and potentially preventable health problems, specific possible types of intervention, research needs, and other activities, but it does not prescribe a federally designed blueprint. Indeed, the country is not a homogeneous political, economic, and social community. Needs and possible solutions to problems could and should be different, as are contrasting areas such as Washington, D.C.; Reno, Nevada; and Aroostook County, Maine. In any initiative it would seem prudent and appropriate to relate programs to regional and local experience.

The secretary, in his preface to the report, states its purpose to be that of encouraging a "second public-health revolution." The first he characterizes as the struggle against infectious diseases, its principal strategies being improved sanitation and immunization. The second revolution is directed toward the less etiologically discrete entities, such as cardiovascular disease, cancer, and accidents. Their causes are more extensively rooted in a variety of social problems, lifestyles, and environmental hazards. To deal effectively with these problems requires a new generation of health professionals. The best of behavioral science and health education will be needed to effect changes in lifestyle. Important contributions will also be made by those engaged in public information, marketing, and merchandising, because the promotion of less-hazardous activity and practice is ultimately more effective than moralistic injunction; from those who market Coca Cola, McDonald's hamburgers, and Fuller brushes we have a lot to learn. Environmental problems increasingly require physical scientists—toxicologists, physicists, and chemists. Since changes in public policy—whether in the area of synthetic fuel development or pesticide use—have major implications for health and for the economy; economists, political scientists, experts in public policy, and lawyers inevitably will play a more central role. With its expanded horizons, the practice of preventive medicine and public health over the coming decades will undoubtedly assume a character quite different from the past and will extend its boundaries far beyond the traditional confines of curative medicine. The major advances will be pioneered and the soundest judgments rendered by those with a multidisciplinary background of education and experience.

The focusing of the surgeon general's report on the developing stages of a "second revolution"—or the need for specific programs in disease prevention and health promotion—is timely and cogent. Implicit is the evolution of preventive medicine and public health from its past role as essentially a medical subspecialty into a unique field of endeavor that embraces not only medical specialists but many others as well. The hour, however, is late, and action is imperative.

HEALTHY PEOPLE: THE SURGEON GENERAL'S REPORT AND THE PROSPECTS

Lawrence W. Green, Dr. P.H.
Director, Office of Health Information, Health Promotion and Physical Fitness, U.S. Department of Health and Human Services

On the same day in October that smallpox was officially declared an eradicated disease, the Public Health Service (PHS) released the final printing of *Healthy People: The Surgeon General's Report on Health Promotion and Disease Prevention* (Department of Health, Education and Welfare 1979b). This is one country's response to the new impetus described by D. A. Henderson (1979). The thesis of this report, in a sentence, is that if the United States is to improve the health of its citizens appreciably in the years ahead, it must reorder its present priorities in health care to put greater emphasis than ever before on the prevention of disease and the promotion of health in people other than patients and with methods other than medical.

Health as a positive concept responds to the new challenge signaled by the eradication of one of the most dreaded infectious diseases. Degenerative diseases—chief among them heart disease, cancer, and stroke—have largely replaced infectious and communicable diseases as the principal threats to life and health. Chronic, degenerative diseases now account for 75 percent of all deaths in this country each year. We are learning that, to a great extent, these diseases, too, can be prevented, but with a quite different set of public health strategies from those deployed in the infectious era.

The most frequent causes of death among individuals between the ages of one and forty are called accidents. Annually, some 100,000 Americans die in situations referred to as accidents, half of them on the highways. An accident, by definition, cannot be prevented, but circumstances that are associated with accidents can be avoided. Injuries and disability can be prevented. Most of the deaths and much of the disability associated with accidents need not occur.

Environmental hazards, in the air we breathe and in the water we drink, at home, at play, and on the job, exact an unnecessarily high toll on our health. There may be only so much that individuals, acting alone, can do about many of these often complex problems, but by working together, Americans can improve the quality of their environments, and consequently of their health.

Behavior of the more personal and private variety contributes enormously to many of our most serious health problems. For example, about 350,000 people die each year from diseases directly linked to cigarette smoking. Another 200,000 deaths, including many of the accidents that take such a heavy toll on younger Americans, are related to the misuse of alcohol. Unhealthy habits can be changed, just as surely as environmental hazards, accidental injuries, and chronic diseases—the chief threats to health today—can be ameliorated, controlled, or otherwise prevented. Experts now are convinced that the reduction of risk and the adoption of positive health practices hold the keys to better health in the years ahead. "Further improvements in the health of the American people can and will be achieved," the surgeon general's report states, "not alone through increased medical care and greater health expenditures, but through a renewed national commitment to efforts designed to prevent disease and to promote health" (DHEW 1979b: 9).

Support from the American people for these shifting priorities in health appears to be positive. The surgeon general's report was released with a minimum of fanfare—no news conference, not even a press release. The first printing of 2,000 copies was simply mailed out, to federal, state, and local health personnel, for the most part, and also to members of the working press. Yet, the following day, newspapers in all parts of the country featured release of the report prominently. The *Wall Street Journal, Los Angeles Times, Boston Globe, Atlanta Constitution, Chicago Sun-Times,* and *New York Daily News* all gave this story front- and second-page coverage.

The health care and health education communities cannot help but be encouraged by the fact that so many leading newspapers, which in their selection and placement of articles reflect the interests and concerns of their readers, elected to give such prominent coverage to a government report on disease prevention and health promotion. Clearly the subject has a special appeal to the American people.

The shape of health care in this country has been changing for some time, and a front-page prevention story, the uniqueness of its appearance notwithstanding, is neither the first nor the most important piece of corroborating evidence. Americans, as the report has documented, are healthier today than ever before. Our infant mortality rate is at its lowest point in history: 13.6 per 1,000 live births. Our people are living longer. The average span of life is now 73.2 years—up 2.7 years in the last decade alone.

The major communicable diseases no longer figure substantially in mortality tables. Some of the chronic diseases that have supplanted them are in retreat, as well. Over the past ten years, for example, deaths from cardiovascular disease have dropped 22 percent. By the time today's children reach adulthood, heart and circulatory diseases may no longer pose major threats to life and health.

It is evident that many of our recent gains in health status can be attributed to actions that people have been taking to help themselves and to measures that communities have been taking to protect their citizens. Over the past several years, this country has witnessed an evolutionary change in national thinking about the protection and enhancement of personal health. As the American people have grown increasingly health-conscious, so have they come to realize the extent to which their physical and emotional well-being depends upon preventive health measures, many of which they, themselves, can effect.

The prevention of heart disease is a case in point. Although epidemiologists are reluctant to ascribe the ten-year decline in heart disease deaths to precise causes, they do point out that cigarette smoking, high blood pressure, and elevated serum cholesterol—three major risk factors that can be influenced, either wholly or in part, by individual action—also declined during this same period.

Health professionals, too, have begun to renew their confidence in methods other than medical and surgical for health care. Increasingly, they have been devoting their time and their talents to activities that can help their patients and communities forestall the onset of disease and achieve healthier, more productive lives. And they have been attending in greater numbers and with more telling effect to problems in the social and physical environments in which their patients live and work.

Healthy People is a reflection, or perhaps, even better, a product, of both the solid record of progress that American medicine and public health have achieved and of our society's growing interest in health as a positive concept. But it is far from a final product or end in itself. Rather, it is one part of a logical process that the Department of Health and Human Services and the Public Health Service have initiated, a process that has as *its* end point the development of a coherent national policy for the prevention of disease and the promotion of good health.

The formal policy development process began in December 1977, when a task force composed of representatives of all HEW agencies was convened to take inventory and to analyze federal programs in disease prevention and health promotion. The report of this body, chaired by Dr. J. Michael McGinnis, was released in September 1978. In addition to comment on existing programs, it also provided a conceptual framework for prevention and recommended a set of strategies for health promotion and disease prevention for action by the federal government.

This document—*the Report of the Departmental Task Force on Prevention* (DHEW 1979a)—figured importantly in the preparation of the surgeon general's report. So, too, did a collection of background papers on prevention and health promotion that was produced, at the request of the surgeon general, by the National Academy of Sciences Institute of Medicine (1979).

The surgeon general's report itself was prepared by the Public Health Service, under the direction of Dr. McGinnis, assisted by a number of other federal agencies and in close collaboration with scientists and health educators from outside government, together with state and local officials, business and labor leaders, representatives of voluntary organizations, and many others.

Most serious illnesses, the report makes clear, are related to not one, but several, risk factors. Some of these risks, such as cigarette smoking, poor dietary habits, and severe emotional stress, have been implicated in the development of several illnesses. Moreover, the combined potential for harm of many risk factors is always greater than the sum of their individual potentials, because they interact with, reinforce, and even multiply each other.

"It is the controllability of many risks," the report concludes, "and often the significance of controlling even a few, that lies at the heart of disease prevention and health promotion" (DHEW 1979b).

Accordingly, the report focuses on the major health problems and their associated risks at each of the five principal stages of life, and it presents a quantified goal, to be achieved by the year 1990, for each stage. The stages examined by the report are infancy, childhood, adolescence and young adulthood, adulthood, and older adulthood. The goals selected for each stage, as outlined in Dean Henderson's paper, are based on recent U.S. mortality trends, rates achieved by other countries that have resources similar to those of the United States, and, in the words of the report, "the very great likelihood that a reasonable, affordable effort can make the goals achievable" (DHEW 1979b).

The report also enumerates fifteen priority "actions for health" that experts believe will be critical to the achievement of the five major goals. These activities are grouped in three overlapping categories:

1. Preventive health services, including family planning, pregnancy and infant care, immunizations, sexually transmissible diseases services, and high blood pressure control, which are normally delivered to individuals by health providers
2. Health protection measures, including toxic agent control, occupational safety and health, accidental injury control, infectious agent control, and fluoridation of community

water supplies, which can be taken by governmental and other agencies, as well as by industry, to protect people from harm

3. Health promotion efforts, including smoking prevention, reducing misuse of alcohol and drugs, improved nutrition, exercise, and stress management, which individuals and communities can undertake to promote changes in behavior and in the social and economic environment to support improvements in health

These fifteen programs or actions were selected from recommendations made by a number of PHS-sponsored working groups. Although the deliberations of these groups were national in perspective, the priorities that emerged are flexible, in the sense that they may be modified to meet local health needs and conditions. In order to provide a base for each action for health from which could be developed a carefully considered plan for carrying it out and for measuring the success or failure of the effort, the next step in the policy development process was undertaken.

In June of 1979, experts from all parts of the country were called to an HEW-sponsored conference in Atlanta to assist in the drafting of measurable objectives for each of the fifteen target areas. These objectives were far more specific and detailed than those in the surgeon general's report. As a sign that the development of prevention policy really is moving forward in an organized and logical way, it is noteworthy that this conference was convened well before the release of the report. Thus, in early August, even as *Healthy People* was coming off the press, HEW was distributing draft objectives from the conference, for comment and review, to some 3,000 individuals and organizations outside the department, as well as to HEW headquarters units and regional offices (Office of Health Information and Health Promotion 1979a).

The final objectives, which will take into account all comments received, will be consistent with the National Health Planning Guidelines, developed by the Health Resources Administration, and the Model Standards for Community Preventive Health Services, developed by the Center for Disease Control. When complete, these objectives will provide a frame-

Figure 3-1. Planning for Disease Prevention and Health Promotion

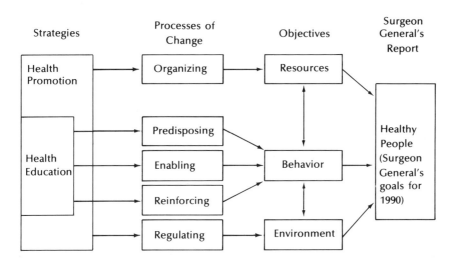

work for all our efforts to improve health over the next decade. Current plans call for releasing them to the public sometime in 1980 at a national conference of leaders from across the country who can stimulate and guide action in the communities to prevent disease and promote health. The relationships among these steps are suggested in Figure 1.

The Public Health Service is moving ahead to implement the recommendations of the surgeon general's report and to prepare for the eventual initiation of the measurable objectives. A most important concern, right now, is the development of a tracking system, which should be in place by the time the objectives are fully developed and which will be employed to plot the evolution of programs and the achievement of goals through 1990 and beyond. Each of the six Public Health Service agencies has been participating in this effort; each has been working, as well, to strengthen its prevention programs.

The Health Resources Administration, for example, has been a valuable partner in the development of prevention objectives and has been taking steps to improve the prevention capabilities of Health Systems Agencies.

The National Institutes of Health last year determined that $350 million of their total research budget was being spent on primary prevention studies, with large proportions devoted to research on reduction of cardiovascular risks and investigations of the toxic effects of pesticides, asbestos, and petrochemicals.

The Alcohol, Drug Abuse, and Mental Health Administration has had three legislatively mandated priorities—services, research, and training. Prevention has now been made a fourth priority. In September, ADAMHA hosted a conference— The First Annual Conference on Prevention—designed to open a dialogue with state and local leaders on issues related to the prevention of alcohol and drug abuse, and to mental health problems. Most of these issues relate to health education of the public and of professionals dealing with the public.

The Center for Disease Control (CDC) has served as a principal prevention agency, conducting epidemiological research related to chronic diseases and to occupational safety and health, providing preventive health and risk reduction services through its grant programs and developing model school health education curricula. The Public Health Service is now considering measures to strengthen CDC's ability to serve as a leading prevention agency.

The Public Health Service also has established a National Health Promotion Program, which is operated by the Office of Health Information, Health Promotion, and Physical Fitness (OHP). This program has sponsored a series of regional forums on community health promotion (OHP 1979b); it also has conducted a program of technical assistance to community health promotion programs. But in terms of increasing public awareness of the benefits of disease prevention and health promotion, two of its most important responsibilities may prove to be the new National Health Information Clearinghouse (NHIC), which was mandated by Title XVII of the Public Health Service Act, and the National Health Promotion Media Campaign, slated to get underway in 1980.

During its first year, the NHIC will be developing its capacity to respond to public inquiries, generally, and especially those that the media campaign generates. In this way, the campaign and the clearinghouse will serve complementary functions, the campaign helping to introduce the clearinghouse to the public as a valuable information resource and the clearinghouse assisting in a vital aspect of the campaign—the distribution of materials. Because the OHP is committed to the decentralization of health promotion initiatives, the clearinghouse will refer as many inquiries, of all kinds, as it can to appropriate federal, state, regional, and local agencies.

The overall goal of the National Health Promotion Media Campaign is to increase public awareness of actions that individuals can take, alone and in concert with others, to maintain and improve their health. The campaign's primary messages— to be communicated in television and radio public-service announcements, newspaper and magazine advertisements, and on posters and transit cards—are that health risks differ from person to person, in kind and degree, and that individuals can take steps to identify and reduce or eliminate the risks most likely to threaten their own health (Green 1979b).

Campaign materials will introduce the concept of *relative* risk and will encourage people to write to the clearinghouse for an OHP-prepared booklet that will feature a self-scoring, risk assessment test. The booklet will provide general information on ways to reduce the risks that readers have discovered by taking the test, and it will tell where and how to obtain more detailed health-risk appraisals. It will also advertise two more booklets that will be available from the NHIC and other sources. One will describe actions that citizens can take, collectively, to address neighborhood and community health promotion issues and concerns. The other will list possible sources of funding for community health promotion activities (Green 1979a).

The initiatives underscore the fact that every programmatic action in the field of disease prevention and health maintenance, every new step, must be based on a foundation of knowledge that is scientifically sound but often not conclusive. Continued research is needed to strengthen that foundation. Breakthroughs in research related to prevention, throughout the history of public health, usually have preceded improvements in health and well-being. Advances in knowledge about nutrition, sanitation, and immunization have brought about reductions in most infectious diseases. A better understanding of the roles of high blood pressure, smoking, and nutrition has enabled us to reduce deaths from heart disease and stroke.

A great deal remains to be learned, of course. We need to know more about the role of toxic substances in the development of chronic diseases and the effects on health of diet and behavior. We need to find more-effective ways of enhancing healthy behavior, and newer and better ways of delivering preventive services (Green 1978). As one indication of our society's commitment to both the pursuit and the application of these kinds of knowledge, it should be noted that the department's fiscal year 1980 budget proposals to Congress reflected an increase in spending for prevention of about $150 million over the 1979 level. And the chances are good that another increase will be requested for FY 1981.

The correlation between suboptimal health and the conditions in which people live is well known. The availability or absence of such necessities as food, jobs, shelter, and medical care exert powerful influences on growth and development at all stages of life.

In these circumstances, unilateral intervention is of little avail. Medical care alone, for instance, will not substantially alter the impact of chronic disease and disability among the disadvantaged, nor will it effectively reduce infant mortality and morbidity. Economic development and health, the direction-general of the World Health Organization has observed, are indivisible.

The expectations of success that we have for programs in disease prevention and health promotion must be geared to this reality. They must capture the attention of all concerned citizens, public and private, and focus it with meaningful effect on what might properly be called the environmental problems of the poor. Moreover, because poor health is the most serious manifestation of these problems, the public health professions must be prepared to lead and, indeed, advance the issue, by strengthening the preventive components of programs already in place, by designing and implementing more innovative efforts, and by serving, across the board, as advocates for the poor.

Obstacles exist on other fronts, too, and predominant among them, perhaps, is the reluctance of many individuals to adopt more healthful patterns of behavior. Although opinion polls note increased interest in health, too many Americans remain unmoved, apparently convinced that illness is an event over which they have no control. Some of these same individuals, including many health professionals, question the scientific validity of programs to promote health. They prefer to stand pat, to wait for more evidence to come in. We still have a great deal to learn, they say.

In this last respect, at least, they are right. For the fact is that we do not know all there is to know about personal health practices and their impact on physical and emotional well-being. We *do* still have much to learn. But no longer, we have come to understand—and this is the big change that has taken place in recent years—no longer can we afford to be hesitant about promoting those practices that we believe to be beneficial or about taking action against those that we suspect may be harmful, simply because we lack every last piece of corroborating scientific evidence. In an imperfect world, we cannot wait for perfect solutions. We must work with what we have, and the time to begin is now.

Personal lifestyles are responsible for much of the unnecessary disease and disability in the United States today. As former HEW Secretary Joseph Califano put it in his foreword to the surgeon general's report, "You, the individual, can do more for your own health and well-being than any doctor, any hospital, any drug, any exotic medical device" (DHEW 1979b).

If responsibility for good health begins with the individual, it extends from there to others in the family and even in the community. The role of exemplar is at once obvious and of critical importance for the parent who is helping to shape the health practices of a coming generation. By participating in community efforts to ensure the availability of appropriate health services and recreational facilities and by encouraging the development of sound health curricula in the schools, adults of all ages can enhance their own health and that of their families, and the quality of life in their community.

Given the benefits that accrue to everyone when people take an enlightened and active interest in their own health destiny, the processes by which these benefits are achieved deserve strong societal support. Most of these processes will require health education. Many people are aware of the implications, good and bad, of personal health behavior, but their readiness to act on that knowledge quite often is lacking. To help people confront the consequences of their personal choices, to develop and make available the methods and support systems that will help them change behavior that should be changed—these are educational and organizational responsibilities that all elements of our society must share. If we are to succeed in our efforts to prevent disease and promote even higher levels of health, we will do so together or, most likely, not at all.

Health professionals have a special obligation to provide people with information that will predispose them, resources and skills that will enable them, and encouragement that will reinforce them in their efforts to deal with behavior they are trying to change. The advice and counsel that citizens receive from those who know the subject best will equip them to assume more and more responsibility for their own health, and it will make them able to use medical services more appropriately at times of injury and illness. Patients *do* listen to their physicians; people *do* want to learn more about safeguarding their health. Physicians, nurses, dentists, and other health professionals must be trained and must come to think of themselves not only as practitioners of particular disciplines but as educators and role models, as well (Green 1979c).

Communities have tremendous resources for fostering disease prevention and health promotion, ranging from voluntary agencies and civic groups to religious organizations and local media. The keys to employing these resources effectively are leadership, careful planning, coordination, and creativity. The objectives, in all cases, should be to provide useful services and to create a climate of interest in better health (Tompkins forthcoming).

With more than 40 million youngsters in school today, teachers are in a better position than any other community group to help our youngest citizens make sound decisions about health—decisions that, in all likelihood, will set lifelong patterns of behavior. This is why comprehensive school health education activities, which foster knowledge and sharpen a child's decisionmaking skills, are so vitally important. They pay dividends today in shares of better health, and for years, even generations, to come (Bureau of Health Education 1977; Castile and Jerrick 1979).

In every community, of course, the work site provides an appropriate—increasingly, a *necessary*—setting for both health promotion and health protection activities. A number of companies today provide physical fitness programs for employees, and in many cases these programs quite literally are paying for themselves in terms of improved employee morale and corporate public relations, but particularly from the savings that accrue when increased numbers of workers remain healthy, productive, and on the job (McGill 1979).

Although it is true that individuals can do much to reduce their own risks of disease, the steps they take in this direction do not, in and of themselves, constitute a comprehensive strategy for preventing illness and for protecting and promoting health. The equation is not that simple; it includes too many factors over which individuals have little or no control.

When problems in disease prevention and health protection cannot be alleviated by individual action or by traditional medical means, the greater resources of society—primarily government, often at all levels—must be marshaled, first to quantify the threat to health and then to protect the largest possible number of citizens from harm.

This pattern of intervention is at once appropriate and familiar in our pluralistic system of delivering health care. Federal and state governments have wide-ranging responsibilities in disease prevention and health promotion. They pay the bills for many services delivered, through such programs as Medicare and Medicaid. They provide leadership in the setting of prevention priorities and goals. They conduct basic research and data collection, and they determine and enforce health and safety standards.

The contributions of local governmental units to the success of prevention programs are no less important. Sanitation measures, water purification, surveillance and control of epidemics—all are, and have been, community concerns. Local laws and ordinances requiring immunization as a prerequisite to school attendance have been instrumental in the success of the National Childhood Immunization Initiative. Fluoridation of community water supplies has been called a primary factor in the relatively high levels of dental health that the American people enjoy today.

The diversification of responsibility for disease prevention and health promotion—a diversification that begins with the individual and encompasses every element of society—is both necessary and desirable. Good health is everyone's concern.

What has been lacking up to now, however, the surgeon general's report points out in its closing pages, has been a mechanism for coordinating these various elements and for giving focus and direction to the new opportunities and approaches that have emerged. If good health has been everyone's concern, it also has been no one's primary responsibility. Health educators and some progressive public health, medical, and nursing professionals have attempted to provide leadership, but with limited support.

However, times are changing. Our ability to link and coordinate the resources available at different levels grows stronger daily, as governors, county officials, and mayors come to grips with the new needs in prevention. They know that by helping each other they can best help themselves and their constituencies.

The 205 newly created health systems agencies and state health-planning bodies provide not only a means of responding to the needs of their respective populations by a national network that can give form and substance to our changing view of good health and of the ways in which it can best be achieved and maintained.

At stake here, as noted by Dean Henderson, is the development of a coherent national policy for the prevention of disease and the promotion of good health. It will take time to construct this policy— to assemble the myriad pieces and to bring together the disparate, often conflicting, points of view that will have to be reconciled if our efforts are to succeed. But with the publication of the surgeon general's report, which indicates so clearly both the challenges and the opportunities that lie ahead, the men and women of the Public Health Service have signified their determination to begin. Some parts of the private sector were already there, notably the Blue Cross and Blue Shield Plans.

If commitments are made at every level of the public and private sectors, the report concludes, "we ought to attain the goals established in this report, and Americans who might otherwise have suffered disease and disability will instead be healthy people."

References

Bureau of Health Education, Center for Disease Control, 1977. *The School Health Curriculum Project* (December). Atlanta, Ga.: BHE/CDC.

Castile, A. S., and S. J. Jerrick, 1979. *School Health in America: A Survey of State School Health Programs.* 2d ed. (August). Atlanta, Ga.: Bureau of Health Education, Center for Disease Control.

Department of Health, Education and Welfare. 1979a. *Disease Prevention & Health Promotion: Federal Programs and Prospects—Report of the Departmental Task Force on Prevention, September 1978.* Washington, D.C.: Government Printing Office.

Healthy People: The Surgeon General's Report on Health Promotion and Disease Prevention. (DHEW Pub. no. 7955071). Washington, D.C.: Government Printing Office.

Green, L. W. 1978. "Determining the Impact and Effectiveness of Health Education as It Relates to Federal Policy." *Health Education Monographs* 6 (suppl. 1).

———.1979a. "Health Promotion Policy and the Placement of Responsibility for Personal Health Care." *Family and Community Health* 2.

———.1979b. "National Policy in the Promotion of Health." *International Journal of Health Education* 22.

———.1979c. "Toward National Policy for Health Education." In *Youth, Alcohol, and Social Policy,* edited by H. T. Blane and M. E. Chafetz. New York: Plenum Publishing Co.

Henderson, D. A. 1979. "Prevention and Public Health." Paper presented at the Blue Cross-Blue Shield 50th Anniversary Symposium, Washington, D.C., December 11-12.

McGill, A. M., ed. 1979. *Proceedings of the National Conference on Health Promotion Programs in Occupational Settings.* Washington, D.C.: Office of Health Information and Health Promotion.

National Academy of Sciences, Institute of Medicine. 1979. *Healthy People: The Surgeon General's Report on Health Promotion and Disease Prevention—vol. 2: Background Papers.* Washington, D.C.: Government Printing Office.

Office of Health Information and Health Promotion. 1979a. *Promoting Health/Preventing Disease: Objectives for the Nation.* Drafts from the Atlanta Conference for Review and Comment (August). Washington, D.C.: OHP.

———.1979b. *Promoting Health: Issues and Strategies.* Washington, D.C.: OHP.

Tompkins, G. Forthcoming. *Organizing Events for Community Health Promotion.* Washington, D.C.: Office of Health Information and Health Promotion.

HEALTH PROMOTION AS PUBLIC POLICY: THE NEED FOR MORAL GROUNDING

Edmund D. Pellegrino, M.D.
President, Catholic University of America

The promotion of health was a central tenet of Hippocratic medicine and of Paidea, the Greek educational ideal (Jaeger 1944). Today, in the midst of the golden age of curative medicine, the time of this ancient ideal seems to have come again. There are mounting pleas for extensive national programs of prevention and health promotion. They promise to compete for expenditures with curative medicine. A public debate over the allocation of funds is in the offing.

The debate will focus on the choices between beneficial options, such as cure and prevention, or personal freedoms and the social and economic welfare of the nation. It will turn on such questions as the allocation of scarce resources, the potential conflict of individual and social good, and the extent to which even the most benign government may intervene in our personal lives to improve our health habits (Wikler 1978).

These are moral questions not to be settled on economic and political grounds alone. They involve our conceptions of the good life. Their resolution requires some moral principles against which to measure conflicting goals and obligations. An ethics of preventive medicine and health promotion is part of the expansion of ethical concerns to include a broad range of health-related public-policy decisions (Tancredi 1974; Outka 1974).

No formal ethics of prevention is currently at hand to set the normative guidelines for the forthcoming debate. This essay offers some tentative principles that might ground the choices. It is tentative and sketchily developed, but I hope only to underscore the need for a more formal and fully developed ethics of prevention.

Dr. Henderson's paper and the surgeon general's report of July 1979 (Department of Health, Education and Welfare

1979), urge us to take action as a nation to modify drastically our personal behavior. They point out, as did the Lalonde report of a few years ago (1974), that billions of dollars could be saved if we eliminate smoking, control obesity, curb alcohol and drug use, modify work and living environments, drive safely, exercise regularly, and cope reasonably with emotional stress. They confirm, too, that the cumulative effects of medical cures on national health are small compared to what could be accomplished by more-hygienic living (McKeown 1979).

Aristotle's conviction that the good society is not possible without healthy citizens seems to be capturing human imagination once again. Unlike the ancients, however, we are motivated by the enormous economic burdens of unhygienic lifestyles rather than the inherent good of a healthy life or its necessity for the good society. We live in a more organized and interdependent society in which individual actions may quickly touch the lives and pocketbooks of others. Our solutions must be on a national, and ultimately, an international scale. They must go beyond the obvious measures of sanitation, quarantine, and immunization. Their success depends upon massive changes in personal behavior—and on an energetic pursuit of the public health.

However, our national experiences with the energy and environmental crises, with gun control and crime, show all too painfully our collective proclivity for short-term satisfactions over long-term social benefits. To modify personal health habits, therefore, implies not only some effective form of persuasion but even some coercion in selected instances. The proposed measures range from the mildest kinds of coercion, like education and opinion manipulation through the mass media, to the more forceful, like tax- and insurance-dollar incentives and disincentives, to the most coercive—legal prohibition.

The social and moral implications of these proposed measures are of the utmost significance in a democratic and pluralistic society. They touch on the kind of life we think worth living, on the things we are willing to trade for good health and economic security, on the balance between libertarian autonomy and government dictates. There is unlikely to be universal consensus on these matters in a democratic society that promises a maximal degree of personal choice. Yet we must define what constraints, if any, we can accept to enhance the common good, which promises to elude us unless we do alter our deleterious lifestyles.

The debate promises to be as difficult as it is indispensable. There are true believers on all sides of the question—some who see health as a new salvation theme for mankind, others who would willingly run the risks of bodily damage and economic disaster so they can pursue their own version of the good life, however harmful it may be. Still others place fiscal and economic health as the first needs of a good society and convert economics into ideology (Pellegrino in press).

The line of argument that is, and will be, debated is simple enough: Certain lifestyles result in disease, disability, and death, with economic consequences damaging to the whole of society. There is, therefore, a social mandate to encourage healthier lifestyles in all citizens. But completely voluntary measures promise to be ineffective. Therefore, for the good of all, measures to enforce personal compliance are justified.

This line of argument is customarily advanced or attacked on economic and political grounds because these aspects are more familiar and urgent to decisionmakers than moral discourse. Granting their obvious importance, economic and political philosophies are themselves founded on more fundamental human values, and these must be more explicitly examined if moral choices are to be made among policy alternatives.

If the forthcoming debates about health promotion are to be based more firmly, two things are required at a minimum: (1) Whatever measures are selected for universal application must be demonstrably effective, which is to say that the probability of success must be high enough to warrant making difficult choices among competing good things, and (2) The choices themselves must rest on some set of explicit moral principles. I cannot do more here than outline what I mean by these two conditions for a morally grounded public-policy debate.

Debates about the ethical use of new knowledge or techniques often go awry because of unrecognized uncertainties in the data supporting their application. To distinguish what is known with certainty, what is unknown, and what is problematic is admittedly difficult, but it is the first step in any debate. Experts who are the guardians of "the facts" all too often are "true believers" and are easily tempted to screen out uncertainties in their favored technique or to confuse technical with moral authority.

But experts have no special prerogatives entitling them to make value judgments for the rest of humankind. Their discretionary space is necessarily limited (Pellegrino 1977). Their unique responsibility is to provide valid fact statements and to outline alternatives. Only in this way can the moral implications of different decisions be properly weighed. Policymakers and moralists working with uncertain facts can go dangerously and foolishly astray.

With respect to health promotion there are two preeminent fact questions in deciding whether a proposed modification of personal behavior is morally defensible: (1) How good is the causal connection between the suspect behavior and disease? And (2), does the method proposed to modify deleterious behavior actually do so? Decisions about the justifiability of a preventive measure or a method of changing behavior must start with reliable facts about causal connection and effectiveness.

The usefulness of preventive measures and advisability of their widespread promotion depend on the strength of the evidence linking certain personal habits to specific illnesses. Some of the relationships are firmly established, others are suggestive but not proven, and others merely speculative.[a]

For example, there is no doubt now that smoking causes coronary disease, emphysema, and cancer of the lung, larynx, esophagus, tongue, and lip; that alcohol is linked to cirrhosis and automobile and airplane accidents, and, coupled with smoking, increases the incidence of laryngeal and esophageal cancers; that caries is linked to carbohydrates in the diet; that salt and hypertension, obesity, and increased morbidity go hand in hand; that asbestos, radiation, and certain industrial chemicals are linked to cancer; that early multiple sexual contacts and herpes simplex viruses are linked to cancer of the

---

[a] No attempt is made here to cite the voluminous literature supporting these statements, and a special case is not being made for the classification. What is essential is that there are varying degrees of certitude as to causation and in each instance that degree must be ascertained as precisely as possible, or moral implications cannot be correctly weighed.

cervix; that higher auto speeds, and driving without seat belts (or a motorcyclist's driving without a helmet) are associated with fatal accidents. In these instances the evidence is direct and obtained from observations in humans.

In other examples, the evidence is suggestive but not well substantiated, limited to subsets of the population, or obtained in test systems whose congruence with human diseases is uncertain. Here, among others, we might cite saturated fat and cholesterol in the diet, the utility of vigorous exercise, and damaging effects of stress, the relation of the nitrites and cyclamates to cancer, the cost benefits of multiple screening, the importance of dietary fiber content, or the relationships of hard water to coronary disease.

In still other examples, the relationships are speculative and in need of much more study before preventive measures can reasonably be prescribed. Here we might include the evidence linking a wide variety of food additives, chemicals, and drugs to human cancer; or the epidemiological evidence for higher or lower incidences of cancer, coronary disease, or longevity in certain populations where the interactions of genetic, environmental, social, and cultural factors have yet to be separated; or the relationship of certain emotional and attitudinal states to morbidity and mortality; or the highly debatable status of high doses of vitamins C and E in human disease, to mention a few relationships hotly contested.

Where the evidence is very strong, as in the first group, concerted governmental and public programs to urge voluntary compliance and even to apply coercive measures of varying types would seem justifiable. Where the evidence is suggestive but not fully established, public programs should be undertaken with great caution. Involuntary measures would be difficult to defend morally. Prudent advice through education to individuals might be more in order, allowing each person to decide whether he wishes to err on the side of safety, and in how many situations. When the evidence is merely speculative, only information underscoring the uncertainties would be justified. Even this must be done with caution, because if too many common practices or substances are condemned, the public becomes cynical, throws up its hands, and says "everything causes cancer." This becomes an easy excuse for not changing personal habits, even when such changes would be truly effective.

Even if causal relationships are established, personal behavior must be modified as causes indicate if health is to be promoted. However, the same questions must arise about the effectiveness of the methods proposed to bring about a given change in lifestyle.

Education is the most widely used means for eliciting voluntary compliance with recommendations that promote health. Its efficacy is difficult to assess and often dubious. There are few studies with controls that would show that behavioral change is actually the result of educational intervention. Health habits are tightly woven into the fabric of a person's entire life—one's emotional needs; self-image; social, family, and peer pressures; and changing public opinion about what is chic, sophisticated, or "macho." Movements like the current fashion in jogging and running, the increase of smoking in young girls, the cult of leanness, the vegetarian trend, and the one-a-day vitamin craze, arise in complex matrices in which education may play a major, minor, or insignificant role. Changes in smoking habits among the educated may be an exception. But the precise role of education is still difficult to ascertain in determining most lifestyle changes.

Nor is the formal transfer of information about health sufficient. Complementary measures are usually necessary, such as group discussions, clubs, buddy systems, individual and group psychotherapy, follow-up visits, hypnosis, biofeedback, social group reenforcement, or medication. How much these measures contribute, alone and in combination, is still extremely difficult to assess.

Finally, some of the most important factors correlating with health habits are insusceptible to education or behavior modification: marital status, sex, income, social class, family size, geography, race, culture and ethnic identification, or personality type. These are more powerful determinants of response and relapse rates than modifiable factors like information. They are changed only with difficulty and at considerable risk to personal freedom and the character of our entire society.

None of this is to suggest that sophisticated, multimedia educational methods should not be used, but simply that selected combinations of methods are usually necessary. More significantly, however, we must assess critically the effectiveness of causal connections of deleterious habits and the methods proposed to alter them before undertaking expensive national programs. Moreover, it is on these judgments of effectiveness that the more difficult questions of moral justification of coercive measures must depend.

These admonitions are especially pertinent when we recognize that some of the most productive preventive measures have been less than voluntary: dropping the speed limit to fifty-five miles per hour, immunization, fluoridation, childproof medicine bottles, flameproof pajamas, and package labeling, to mention a few. Before committing ourselves to even the mildest coercive measures, we must have reliable data demonstrating their unequivocal efficacy.

Involuntary measures will continue to be needed in specified areas of health promotion. They must be undertaken with a clear perception of the dangers they pose to a democratic society—loss of personal freedom to choose a lifestyle, dependence upon governments to define values and concepts of the good life, and the imposition of cultural homogeneity. Involuntary measures also assume a benign, wise, and responsive government—something history finds singularly rare.

Each time we partition resources for specific ends—let us say health promotion versus curative medicine, or versus housing, security, crime, or protection of environment—we necessarily limit personal choices about what constitutes a good life. And there is the additional question of injustice to those who want and need other good things, like curative medicine, life-support measures, and rehabilitation. The poor are at special risk, for they cannot pay the costs of surtaxes, increased insurance premiums, and other "disincentives." They cannot enjoy the "luxury" of wealthy persons to choose health-damaging habits. Nor must we forget that one person's prudent, healthy diet and exercise are another person's version of hell—or at least purgatory.

Again, these observations are not meant to argue against health promotion or against morally justifiable coercive measures. They do frame the relevant questions that need debate if we seek a national policy based on moral as well as economic and political considerations.

Even though there is not yet any formally developed ethic of prevention and health promotion that might resolve the moral dilemmas raised in this essay and in Daniel Wikler's excellent paper. (1978), some guidelines are needed if the surgeon general's recommendations are to be applied on a national scale. Without them, health promotion is easily susceptible to the extremes of overzealous application by enthusiasts on the one hand and overprompt rejection by libertarians on the other. This is especially so when involuntary measures must be considered. Since I believe the social and economic benefits of prevention and promotion will require some involuntary measures, I will close this essay with some tentative guidelines for the morally justifiable use of enforcement.

The first principle to be observed is that of proportionality. Coercive measures are to be considered only when their effectiveness is undeniable for large numbers of people and when the affecting control extends over a limited sector of life. "The game must be worth the candle." Examples would be such things as immunization, sanitation, limiting carcinogenic food additives, speed limits, helmets for motorcyclists, nutrition for the newborn, fluoridation, and built-in seat belts. The inconvenience of such measures is small, their social benefit is high, and their economic advantages considerable.

Even if a measure meets the test of proportionality it must accommodate as closely as possible the democratic principle of self-determination. Voluntary measures must be clearly inadequate at the outset, or must have failed, before compulsory measures are contemplated. But even when justified, coercion should be of the mildest sort, compatible with achieving the desired change in behavior. To forestall the imposition of involuntary measures, individuals should be assisted to analyze the consequences of deleterious habits so they can see the value choices they must make and can make those choices on the basis of valid information. This is a new realm of moral obligation for health professionals, especially as we move into programs of self-care and personal promotion of health.

There are several corollaries of the obligation to optimize self-determination. For example, inducements should be favored over disincentives, like tax surcharges or increased premiums. Remediable conditions that make choices less than free must be ameliorated as much as possible through education, by restraints on misleading advertisements, reducing peer and group pressures, and treating emotional problems. True education aimed at providing information to enable free choice must be distinguished from subtle use of the media to covertly manipulate decisions, even for good purposes.

When involuntary or coercive measures are unavoidable, they should be limited severely in matters that are private, like sex, family, and personal amusements. Regulation should be confined to actions with direct public impact, lest moralizing take the place of morality. Similarly, restrictions should be placed on those who take deleterious actions and not on the victims of another's unhygienic habits. Those who wish the freedom to choose unhygienic habits like smoking should be restrained by social quarantine from imposing its unesthetic or unhealthy effects upon others in public places, in the presence of infants, or in the workplace. Social quarantines place the restriction where it belongs—on the source of the socially unacceptable behavior. The same would apply to noisemaking and other forms of nonindustrial pollution of the local social environment.

Regulations should always presume in favor of those whose consent cannot be obtained—infants, children, the retarded, and the senile, or those who must work, let us say, in noisy or chemically polluted environments. In general those who are not in the position to decide should be given the benefit of doubt by the legislating of effective measures to promote health in their behalf.

These examples are all simply corollaries of the rule that freedom must be optimized in a civilized and democratic society and is to be limited only when it violates the freedoms of others. In an interdependent society, free acts that, taken cumulatively, have undesirable effects on the national economy or quality of life are subject to justifiable restriction. However, no civilized society can abandon those who have chosen unwisely and fallen victim to the physical and emotional disorders that result from their damaging lifestyles. They must be treated humanely, even though at public expense and even when resources are scarce.

What is suggested here in the most preliminary way are some moral groundings for public policies in health promotion. They obviously do not in themselves constitute an ethic of public health or preventive medicine.

Today's debates about national policies in health care are urgent enough and universal enough in their effects to become paradigms of the value choices we must make in all policy decisions in a democratic and professedly humane society. Our task is a continuous one—to balance equality and efficiency, personal freedom, and social good, but to do so in morally defensible ways.

An ethic of health promotion and disease prevention is but part of an ethic of health care, and both are steps toward a larger enterprise—an ethic of responsible citizenship and moral governance. It is a mark of a civilized society that its citizens can perceive the tensions that conflicting benefits may engender and yet balance them in reasonable and moral ways that avoid the easy seductions and evils of the extremes.

References

Department of Health, Education and Welfare. 1979. *Healthy People: The Surgeon General's Report on Health Promotion and Disease Prevention.* (DHEW Pub. no. 79-55071.) Washington, D.C.: Government Printing Office

Jaeger, W. 1944. *Paidea, the Ideal of Greek Culture,* vol. 3, ch. 1. New York: Oxford University Press.

Lalonde, M. 1974. *A New Perspective on The Health of Canadians.* Ottawa: Government of Canada (April).

McKeown, T. 1979. *The Role of Medicine: Dream, Mirage, or Nemesis?* Princeton, N.J.: Princeton University Press.

Outka, G. 1974. "Social Justice and Equal Access to Health Care." *Journal of Religious Ethics* (Spring).

Pellegrino, E. D. 1977. "The Expansion and Contraction of Discretionary Space," In *Priorities for the Use of Resources in Medicine* (DHEW Pub. no. [NIH] 77-1288) DHEW Fogarty International Center Proceedings 40, Washington, D.C.

————. In Press. "Medical Economics and Medical Ethics: Points of Conflict and Reconciliation" (Abner Calhoun Lecture). *Journal of the Medical Association of Georgia.*

Tancredi, L., ed. 1974. *Ethics of Health Care*. Washington, D.C.: National Academy of Sciences. See especially "Government Decision-making and the Preciousness of Life," Kenneth J. Arrow, and commentaries by Guido Calabresi and Edmund D. Pellegrino, pp. 33-64.

Wikler, D. I. 1978. *Ethical Issues in Governmental Efforts to Promote Health*. Washington, D.C.: National Academy of Sciences.

4 ENVIRONMENTAL FACTORS AND HUMAN HEALTH

Norton Nelson, Ph.D.
Chairman, Department of Environmental
Medicine
New York University

Norton Nelson, Ph.D., is director of the Institute of Environmental Medicine and chairman of the Department of Environmental Medicine at New York University Medical Center, positions he has held since 1954. The group brought together at the Institute by Nelson has been instrumental in leading a series of pioneering and broad attacks on health problems posed by physical and chemical factors in the environment. These problems have ranged from the mode of action at the intracellular level, through development of animal models for reduction of toxicity, to the conduct of epidemiological studies on humans and field studies of the movement of pollutants through air and water. Under his guidance as the Institute's first full-time scientist, the staff has grown to a total of 200, including 60 scientists and 35 full-time faculty. More than 1,000 papers have been published by the Institute in the past two decades covering a broad range of studies relating to the impact of environmental agents on health. Dr. Nelson has served in many local, national, and international groups in his field of activity, including many committees of the National Research Council. He chaired the committee that produced the book-length report, Principles for Evaluating Chemicals in the Environment. *He also guided a number of major national studies on health effects of environmental agents, including a five-year research plan for the National Institute of En-*

vironmental Health Sciences published as Man's Health and the Environment—Some Research Needs, *a study repeated at the request of Congress in 1976–77.*

There has been a dramatic change in health patterns in the United States, as in most industrialized countries, in the last seventy-five years. In 1900 the life expectancy was forty-nine years, now it is approximately seventy-three. In 1900 pneumonia was a major killer, accounting for approximately 250 deaths per 100,000 per year. Now pneumonia is a more modest, although significant, cause of death, accounting for 35 per 100,000. In 1900 tuberculosis was a major threat to people in their late teens and twenties. Currently it is a relatively rare disease. Diarrheal disorders at the turn of the century accounted for 4,000 deaths per 100,000 per year in children under two; today they are approximately 50 per 100,000 (National Institutes of Health, 1976). Immunization has reduced illnesses from such infections as measles, smallpox, whooping cough, and diphtheria. Many of the endocrine disorders that formerly went uncontrolled are now dealt with routinely; diabetes is an example. At the present time cardiovascular diseases are the major killers, although they appear to be declining somewhat. The second killer is cancer.

Although many of these health advances are traceable to specific intervention, especially improved hygienic measures, such as better water supplies, in other cases there is doubt as to how these changes have come about. The work of McKinlay and McKinlay illustrates in Figures 4–1 and 4–2 the relationship of prophylactic and therapeutic measures to the changing mortality patterns. Remarkably, the curves seem to be largely uninfluenced by those measures.

We are now in a totally different health era. With the dwindling of childhood diseases, we now need to be much more concerned about congenitally determined disorders; in the middle and late teen years accidents become a major threat; and in the later decades chronic diseases, especially cardiovascular disease and cancer, are of outstanding concern. In essentially all cases, excepting perhaps the control of endocrine disorders, disease prevention has been the basis for all our major health advances. At this time the challenge is: Can disease

Figure 4–1.   The Fall in the Standardized Death Rate (per 1,000 Population) for Four Common Infectious Diseases in Relation to Specific Medical Measures, for the United States, 1900–1973

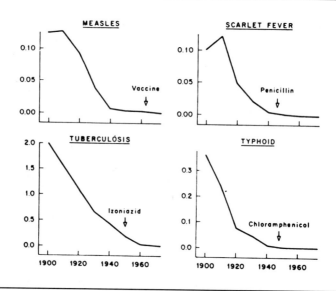

Source: McKinlay, J. B., and S. M. McKinlay. 1977. "The Questionable Contribution of Medical Measures to the Decline of Mortality in the United States in the Twentieth Century." *Millbank Memorial Fund Quarterly* 55:405–428.

prevention decrease the likelihood of congenital disorders and early developmental problems in childhood, extend lifespan, even modestly, or—more important—improve the quality of life and reduce needless suffering?

It will be useful at this point to examine the strategy of prevention and to identify some major difficulties and limitations. It is overly simple to assume that if one identifies the injurious agent, one can intervene, prevent further exposure, and thereby forestall injury. Only in the case of certain occupational factors is this a generally straightforward, and an operationally successful, approach. In those instances where environmental factors are caused by the release of a contaminant or pollutant, whether one is concerned with air, with food, or with water, in theory at least the only barrier to elimination is the cost of

Figure 4–2.   The Fall in the Standardized Death Rate (per 1,000 Population) for Five Common Infectious Diseases in Relation to Specific Medical Measures, for the United States, 1900–1973

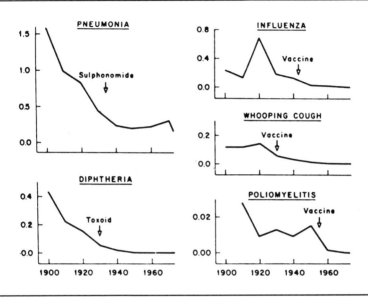

SOURCE: McKinlay, J. B., and S. M. McKinlay. 1977. "The Questionable Contribution of Medical Measures to the Decline of Mortality in the United States in the Twentieth Century." *Millbank Memorial Fund Quarterly* 55:405–428.

preventing release of the pollutant. Sometimes, of course, that cost is excessive, and a point of diminishing returns is reached where expenditures for further control may be relatively ineffective.

However, when one moves into the realm of personal habits, the situation is totally different. Smoking is bad for one's health. Many people who know this very well continue to smoke, finding either that their satisfaction outweighs the risk or, while knowing very well the risks and anxious to stop, they are unable to break the habit. This dilemma is usual with so-called voluntary risks, whose elimination depends on alteration of personal habits. At this stage, prevention moves beyond the domain of the "hard" scientist into that area where behavioral alteration is the only means for success. We have not been very successful in this.

Table 4-1   Chemical and Allied Products Production Index, 1967–1977 (Base: 1967 = 100)

Year	Average Production Index
1967	100.0
1968	109.9
1969	120.4
1970	120.2
1971	126.4
1972	139.3
1976	169.3
Dec. 1977	183.0

SOURCE: Manufacturing Chemists Association. 1973. *Statistical Summary*. Washington, D.C. (Updated from *Chemical Engineering News*, May 1, 1978.)

With this caveat to remind us that identification is not in itself adequate to ensure control of these new breeds of injurious agents, we can move on to examine a series of circumstances that suggest that citizens in this last quarter of the twentieth century are in fact exposed to environmental agents that either are known to be injurious or have sufficient basis of suspicion to require investigation. However, before we proceed to a discussion of environmental factors and disease, let us briefly review growth patterns of technology in this country.

Table 4-1 illustrates the remarkable increase in the production of organic chemicals over the last few decades in the United States. Figure 4-3 shows as one example growth in the production of ethylene (approximately 25 billion pounds annually) and other synthetic organic chemicals. Ethylene is one of the major starting materials for a broad array of synthetic organic chemicals. Chemical technology has now reached the stage where simple molecules from various sources—petrole-

Figure 4–3. Production Trends for Major Petrochemical Starting Materials

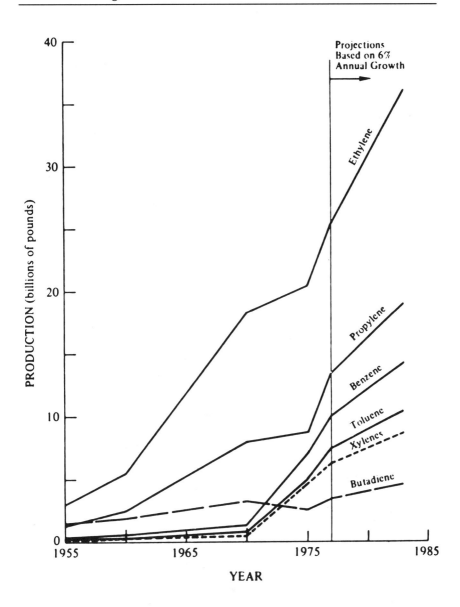

SOURCES: *Science and Tehcnology, A Five Year Outlook,* National Academy of Science, W.H. Freeman and Company, San Francisco, 1979

um, alcohol from fermentation, and others—are converted into a wide variety of products, including the synthesis of other chemicals having many final uses. Some 200 chemicals are now produced annually, in forms that have distributed, or dispersive, noncaptive uses in excess of 25 million pounds per year; 25 of these exceed 100 million pounds per year (President's Biomedical Research Panel 1976). Obviously, most of these chemicals are contained, and the consumer is not exposed; others end up in nontoxic forms. On the other hand, there is generally some loss to the environment. These losses are often regarded as normal and inevitable and may amount to only a small percentage of the total production. However, 1 percent (a conservative estimate of loss prior to the recent imposition of stringent controls) of the 6-billion-pound annual production of vinyl chloride, a known toxic chemical, comes to 60 million pounds. With a fifteen to twenty-five year "incubation" of cancer in heavily exposed workers, effects on large populations of less exposed individuals cannot be assessed in the near future. This is unfortunately true of other environmental agents as well.

Energy production has been until recently growing at an annual rate of 3 to 4 percent. In the last several years it has slowed to about 2 percent, and if the objectives of our national government are fulfilled, it may slow still more. Even with no growth, however, the total energy production in this country is now at a staggering 73×10^{15} BTU per year (Doernberg 1978), equivalent to approximately 8,000 medium power-generating stations. Whether that production is from clean gas, dirty oil, still dirtier coal, or quite clean nuclear energy, some degree of environmental contamination is inevitable.

I would like to review some of the evidence that external, noninfectious agents do contribute to ill health. Some of these suggestions are demonstrated and solid; others remain speculative at this time. In this discussion the terms "environmental" and "external" are used interchangeably to describe noninfectious physical or chemical agents, external to the body, as possible contributors to health impairment. Although most of the hard evidence on the role of external factors comes from occupational exposures, there is a growing body of data suggesting that external factors can play a role in disease and

health impairment in ways unrelated to specific high-level occupational exposures.

There is now no residual doubt that cigarette smoking is a
major source of disease in the United States and many other
parts of the world. Some 80 percent of all lung cancer can be
attributed to cigarette smoking. This amounts to nearly 80,000
deaths per year in this country. In addition, there is good reason to believe that cardiovascular disease is an even more
grave consequence of cigarette smoking, the contribution being
on the order of 225,000 deaths per year (National Institutes of
Health/National Cancer Institute 1978). Cigarette smoking is
also clearly associated with an increased risk of cancer of the
bladder and perhaps other organs as well. There is evidence
that heavy cigarette smoking in expectant mothers may lead
to underweight infants. In certain segments of our population,
drug abuse is also clearly a contributor to ill health and death.

We know, of course, that exposure to chemical and physical
factors in an occupational setting can produce major health impairment and death. Historically, we have had serious worker
disease from exposure to metals such as lead and mercury, and
pneumoconiosis through exposure to silica, coal, and asbestos
particles. Although many workplace contaminants have been
controlled very substantially, especially since new federal regulations have been imposed under the Occupational Safety and
Health Act, nevertheless compliance is far from complete.
Some of the supposedly controlled occupational diseases are
still present and go either undetected or uncontrolled.

The current contribution of occupational exposures to disease and death in this country remains in large degree un-
quantified. Much attention has been given, especially in recent
decades, to cancer from occupational exposure to carcinogenic
chemicals and to ionizing radiation. Indeed, radiologists have
paid a severe penalty for their use of ionizing radiation. As
will be described more fully later, a component of total cancer
from external sources, ranging from as low as 1 to as high as
20 percent or more, has been attributed to occupational exposures (National Cancer Institute et al. 1978).

The production of energy from fossil fuels has received a
great deal of concern for its contribution to community air pollution, and the concern has led to the imposition of substantial

controls. (Now there is the risk that these controls may be relaxed in the present energy crunch.) However, it is generally conceded that community air pollution arising from the combustion of fossil fuels has a significant health impact in increased mortality and morbidity. A report from the National Academy of Sciences concludes that there are annually 15,000 deaths, 7 million illness days spent in bed, and 15 million days of restricted activity, all attributable to air pollution. (National Academy of Sciences/National Research Council 1974). Although the role of air pollution in contributing to cancer—particularly lung cancer—remains in debate, one report attributes the contribution of community air pollution to lung cancer in male cigarette smokers at about 10 percent of the lung cancer incidence in that group (Cederlof et al. 1978). Some disturbance in perception of time and reaction response time are associated with concentrations of carbon monoxide reached in some city streets; still lower levels are associated with the onset of anginal attacks (Environmental Protection Agency [EPA] 1979).

Since effective water treatment has essentially eliminated the danger of infections, water contaminants have been regarded as of relatively minor consequence insofar as human health is concerned. In most instances, water contaminants such as the toxic methyl mercury, a neurotoxin (World Health Organization [WHO] 1976a); polychlorinated biphenyls (PCBs), an animal carcinogen injurious to the fetus (WHO 1976b); and the chlorinated pesticides such as DDT and their metabolites (many of which are animal carcinogens), although present in some potable waters, are found only at low concentrations. However, both methyl mercury and the chlorinated hydrocarbons are bioconcentrated in the food chain in aquatic systems, reaching very substantial levels in fish, and can thus reach man in larger amounts. This has led in each of these instances to the imposition of control measures, including the restriction of sports and commercial fishing in certain areas of the United States. It should be noted that significant amounts of the PCBs and the chlorinated pesticides and their metabolites are widely distributed in the U.S. population in body fat. The fat in human milk shares in this contamination, leading to the consequence that nursing infants are the segment of the population most highly exposed to these compounds (Allen and Barsotti 1976; Savage 1977).

What might be called secondary water contaminants may also be a concern. A number of raw waters being processed for potable supplies contain humic materials in relatively low concentration. In themselves, these are nontoxic; however, during the process of chlorination they react to produce alkyl chlorine compounds, including chloroform. Chloroform has been shown to be carcinogenic in laboratory studies (National Research Council 1977). On this basis, the EPA is moving ahead with a proposal to require cities of over 75,000 population to install charcoal filters in their water systems to remove these organic precursors prior to chlorination (EPA 1978).

Food technology has advanced substantially in the last few decades in improving shelf-life for a variety of products that would not otherwise tolerate transport to widely distributed markets. The Food and Drug Administration has had an excellent record of pretesting such components. Current problems include the nitrites used in the coloring and preservation of meats such as salami, bologna, and wieners. These are of concern in two ways: Nitrite can react in the stomach with secondary amines, producing nitrosamines, which are known potent carcinogens; in addition, recent work suggests that nitrites in themselves may produce cancer in laboratory animals (National Institute of Environmental Health Agencies 1977). There is a move under way at present to reduce nitrite addition substantially.

It should also be mentioned that there are natural toxins in foods which, unlike microorganisms, survive cooking; one of these is aflatoxin, a potent carcinogen. This is a contaminant arising from mold growing on stored seeds and grains. Peanuts appear to be especially prone to such contamination. Aflatoxins are detectable at very low levels and are found normally in peanut butter in this country, but are closely monitored by the Food and Drug Administration. Aflatoxin also may represent one of the first-known instances of a demonstrable dose-response relationship between human cancer and a dietary factor. This observation stems from studies in Africa and southeast Asia associating a greater incidence of cancer of the liver with aflatoxin intake. It may be that this involves interaction with hepatitis infection (Linsell and Peers 1977).

The recent public debate on the saccharin issue is probably not yet settled. There is no question that saccharin is an animal carcinogen and a carcinogen promoter in laboratory studies. The possible impact on humans is not well understood, but there is some epidemiological evidence of measurable elevation of bladder cancer associated with its use (Howe et al. 1977).

Turning to a different area, our concept of the role of some of the heavy metals is changing significantly. Lead, which is now widely distributed throughout the biosphere, is largely there as the result of man's technology. It appears that in primitive and prehistoric times lead concentration in the biosphere was two, or perhaps three, orders of magnitude lower than it is at the present time. A few years ago we were concerned only with acute lead poisoning as observed in children with pica ("licking disease") or workers exposed to high concentrations of lead. It is now evident that body burdens of lead in the so-called normal range may already be at levels at which heme (a constituent of hemoglobin) synthesis is interfered with. There is also some suggestive evidence that these normal or moderately elevated levels may contribute to learning and behavioral difficulties in children (EPA 1977).

Mercury is toxic in itself and becomes very much more toxic when methylated, as it is in the bottom sediments of streams and lakes. As noted earlier, methyl mercury accumulates in the flesh of fish and is thereupon subject to human consumption. Part of the mercury, especially in fresh waters, is man's discharge of mercury. However, mercury has moved through the biosphere in vast quantities for millennia, and it tends to accumulate in fish, especially those living for a long time, such as swordfish (WHO 1976a). Methyl mercury kills neurons, producing acute disease. The concern has been voiced that if methyl mercury continues its toxic effects, it may be contributing significantly at moderate levels of intake to the observed loss of neurons with aging (Weiss and Simon 1975).

Cadmium is known to be a toxin in occupational exposures. Although there is some suggestive evidence of carcinogenicity, of chief interest here is its effect on the kidneys. In occupational exposures, kidney injury is one of the effects observed. Study of normal human tissue shows that cadmium accumulates in the kidneys throughout life, reaching a maximum in the later decades. Cadmium is a ubiquitous constituent of many foods, especially grains, and, although poorly absorbed, is almost totally retained. Thus the newborn infant starts life with a few micrograms of cadmium, but by the decades of the fifties and sixties the body has accumulated a substantial amount, especially in the kidneys and liver. The accumulation in the kidney is in the range, on the average, of one-third of that associated with kidney injury (Friberg et al. 1974). Considering the anticipated variation in patterns of uptake and retention within the normal population, one may speculate that in some instances cadmium may be contributing to the loss of renal function as part of the aging process in some individuals.

There is a finding of some standing, fully meriting attention, that cardiovascular disease is lower in populations consuming hard water than in those consuming less-hard water (National Research Council 1977). These findings, if validated, could justify mineral supplement through deliberate water treatment or other methods aimed at assuring that susceptible populations receive the requisite mineral intake.

Recent findings show that atherosclerotic plaques are of uniform cellular origin—that is, they are monoclonal. Such observations are consistent with their initiation through the mutation of a somatic cell induced by external or internal mutagens (Benditt 1976). Work in the chicken, which has a high rate of atherosclerosis, has shown that the carcinogens/mutagens benzpyrene and dimethylbenzanthracene, when administered to young chickens, accelerate the time of appearance, number, and size of the atherosclerotic plaques (Albert et al. 1977). These findings of an external agent accelerating a pathologic process associated with aging would not eliminate interest in the fats and cholesterol, but would suggest that their role in atherosclerosis should be regarded as an exacerbating, but not initiating, factor.

Another class of problems stems from human exposure to dangerous chemicals through accidents or leaking waste disposal sites. An example of the former was an explosion that scattered dioxin, one of the most toxic chemicals known, over an area around Seveso, Italy (Pocchiari, Silano, and Zampieri 1979). The Love Canal area in the city of Niagara Falls, New York, is an example of large-scale dumping of dangerous waste chemicals in a place where homes and a school were later constructed. Evidence of increased spontaneous abortions and congenital defects among the local population has required large-scale evacuation of the area (New York State Department of Health 1978).

Cancer from external sources has been much in the news recently, and the statement is often made that a large part, perhaps 80 to 90 percent, of cancer is due to external sources. External factors, both chemicals and radiation, can produce cancer. Ultraviolet light has clear association with skin cancer as well as with the genetic constitution of the host (Jablon 1975). We have mentioned occupational cancer, chiefly but not exclusively caused by chemical agents, which is now a well-studied field and one in which new carcinogens continue to be identified as investigations are extended. Thus, within the last ten years a number of new occupational cancer-producing agents have been identified. These include the chloromethyl ethers associated with lung cancer (Nelson 1976); vinyl chloride, associated particularly with angiosarcoma of the liver (Cole and Goldman 1975); epichlorhydrin with lung cancer (Laskin et al. forthcoming); and ethylene oxide with leukemia (Hogstedt, Malmqvist, and Wadman 1979).

There is current debate as to the extent of the contribution of occupation to the total cancer burden in the U.S. population. These estimates range from as low as 1 to as high as 20 percent or more (National Cancer Institute et al. 1978). Part of the disagreement stems from how interaction with other factors is dealt with in such estimates. It is very clear in several instances that cigarette smoking seriously potentiates the effect of exposure to occupational carcinogens; this has been shown for asbestos and lung cancer (International Agency for Research on Cancer 1977) and for the exposure to radon daughter products in uranium mining (U.S. Congress 1969).

There has been apprehension that the growth in chemical technology described earlier may be contributing, or is about to contribute, to a major additional cancer burden on the population. Although there is little data to support this apprehension now, it should be added that all the evidence, because of the long "incubation" period, is not at hand. However, an interesting recent analysis examines age-adjusted cancer mortality by the fraction of population employed in manufacturing enterprise. A rise in the male cancer rate, with increasing percentages for those engaged in manufacturing, is shown in Figure 4–4 when the data are analyzed by state for the United States or internationally in Figure 4–5 by country (Harriss, Hohenemser, and Kates 1978).

Cancer trends over the last five or six decades have shown a major jump in lung cancer, largely attributable to cigarette smoking, but an almost equally dramatic decrease in some other forms of the disease—for example, stomach cancer (Levin et al. 1974). A careful analysis of total cancer rates shows at most a modest annual increase over the last few years (Chiazze, Levin, and Silverman 1977); it is much more instructive to examine cancer rates by organ site. There are, however, grounds for concern rather than complacency. The reality of a number of suggestive trends will be determined only by specific and sharply aimed inquiries, few of which have as yet been undertaken. I cite just one example, based on work of our own institute, which is illustrative of one approach to a more detailed inquiry: On the basis of chemical structure, there are grounds for suspecting that some constituents of hair dyes may be carcinogenic. Short-term bacterial assays showed them to be mutagenic, and, subsequently, long-term tests established the fact that some of these were carcinogenic in rodents (Shore et al. 1979). Because of these suspicions, our epidemiological group undertook a study of a possible relationship between hair dye use and breast cancer. This study (Shore et al. 1979) strongly suggested that there was an association between the intensity and time of use of "permanent" hair dyes and breast cancer (Table 4–2). If these findings are verified, the impact is anything but trivial; an estimate of the impact of hair dye suggests that nearly 3,000 cases of breast cancer per year may be associated with its use. Manufacturers are now changing the composition of these products.

A study of the geographic occurrence of cancer by organ site shows major differences in different parts of the world. Further studies show that migrant populations tend to assume the can-

Figure 4–4.   Cancer mortality rate by state as a percentage of work force engaged in manufacturing

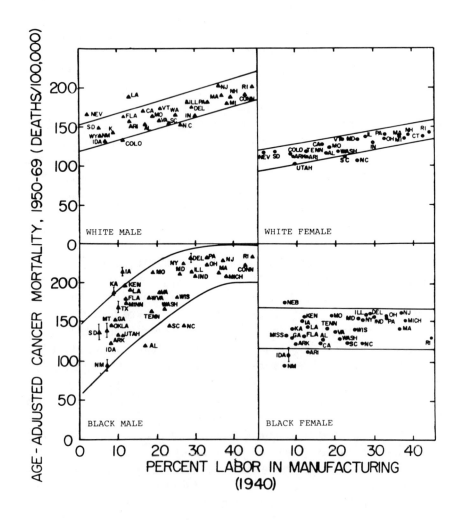

Source Harris, et al, 1978.

Figure 4–5. Cancer mortality rate by country as a percentage of work force engaged in manufacturing

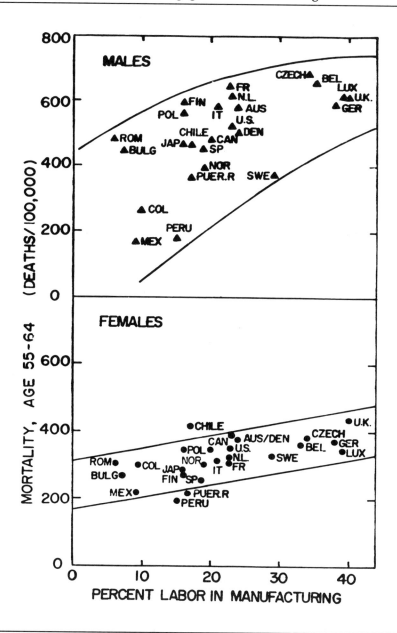

SOURCE Harris, et al, 1978.

Table 4–2   Relative Risks and Integral Use of Hair Colorants Among Breast Cancer and Control Women at Selected Intervals Prior to Breast Cancer

Yrs. Before B-Ca [b]	Adj. Relative Risk [a]	Mean Integral Use		Adj. Trend Tests [a]	
		B-Ca [b]	Cont [c]	Z	(P)
15	1.43	8.7	3.7	2.21	(0.01)
10	1.48	15.4	8.5	2.48	(0.01)
5	1.08	25.6	17.6	1.88	(0.03)
0	1.00	39.4	30.2	1.47	(0.07)

NOTE: Use = frequency × duration.
[a] Adjusted for a Multivariate Index of Risk Factors for Breast Cancer. Trend Tests by Method of Mantel. One-sided P=Values Shown.
[b] B-Ca = Breast Cancer.
[c] Cont = Control.
SOURCES: Courtesy of Dr. Ray Shore, Institute of Environmental Medicine, New York University Medical Center. (See Shore etal., 1979)

cer rate of the region into which they move. Thus stomach cancer is high in Japan, lower in Hawaii in the Japanese migrating there, and still lower among the Japanese in the United States (Haenszel 1975). Similar findings have been found for other organ sites. We are then led to the observation that cancer rates appear to reflect the cultural pattern of the area in which those with cancer live. The term "cultural pattern" is used here to cover a wide range of factors, including diet, personal habits, and occupation, with the probability that diet is an important determinant. The term "lifestyle" has been aptly applied to characterize these observations (Higginson and Muir in press). This wide geographical variation in cancer by organ site, associated with the trend toward assumption of the local cancer pattern by migrants, leads to support the concept that lifestyle or cultural patterns may be determinants of cancer rates by organ site. This is not to imply that genetic factors are unimportant. We know very well that genetic factors play an extremely important role in individual susceptibility to carcinogenic exposures. What it does imply is that the range of genetic variation contributing to host susceptibility, although large, may be roughly the same in different ethnic groups, and that the overwhelming determinant of cancer of particular organs is the cultural pattern into which the migrants move.

Studies such as these have led Higginson and others to speak about the contributions of external factors (e.g., lifestyle, plus smoking, plus occupation) to cancer as being on the order of 80 to 90 percent. These cultural patterns have obviously existed in many places for centuries, and perhaps millennia, and thus bear little relationship to current chemical technology. The question is, do these age-old patterns, especially dietary patterns, determine the different cancer outcomes now found by studies of geographic distribution of cancer? The evidence at this time is highly suggestive that this is the case.

We know very well that cancer from external sources, unlike infectious diseases, is relatively rarely a one-to-one relationship of etiologic agent on the one hand and resultant disease on the other. Even in the high-level exposures associated with industry, interaction is very important. In the case of malignancy in association with cultural patterns, it seems probable that we are concerned here with a complex intermix of carcinogens and promoting, or cocarcinogenic, agents which, acting together, lead to the observed differences in cancer occurrence. In some cases it may be that prevention would be more realistically aimed at control of environmental (or host) enhancing factors rather than a ubiquitous carcinogenic agent. The resolution of this problem will be a challenging scientific endeavor in the next few decades.

There is no question that external noninfectious agents can alter disease patterns in animals and humans. In many of these instances the evidence is still speculative, but it is sufficiently suggestive to merit careful examination. Earlier, the caveat was suggested that identification of causal factors is not equivalent to ability to intervene and successfully prevent exposure. In the complex array of substances and processes discussed here, such intervention will obviously also be a complicated issue. Nevertheless, if these factors are consequential, we need a degree of identification before we can move ahead. Such characterization does not necessarily require that the precise agent or agents be identified—although this would be preferable—but only that the general pattern of living with which the consequences are associated be characterized. Following this will come the search for procedures for intervention, which might take many forms.

It would be wrong to suggest that the gains that await us in this field in the next fifty years can possibly match the dramatic accomplishments of public health, better nutrition, and medical advances of the past seventy-five years. We are not immortal, and miracles will continue to elude us. It seems equally evident, however, that the gain remaining to be achieved is to improve the quality of life throughout the lifespan—that is, to optimize the extent and quality of life to the degree that is realistically achievable. We will continue to die, we hope somewhat later and with less nasty terminal illnesses. Indeed, prolongation of life without improving its quality is no real accomplishment at all. As has been said by someone, "Such prolongation of life might be better described as a prolongation of death."

References

Albert, R. E.; M. Vanderlaan; F. J. Burns; and M. Nishizumi. 1977. "Effect of Carcinogens on Chicken Atherosclerosis." *Cancer Research* 37.

Allen, J. R.; and D. A. Barsotti. 1976. "The Effects of Transplacental and Mammary Movements of PCBs in Infant Rhesus Monkeys." *Toxicology* 6.

Benditt, E. P. 1976. "Implications of the Monoclonal Character of Human Atherosclerotic Plaques." *Annals of the N.Y. Academy of Science* 275.

Cederlof, R.; R. Doll; B. Fowler; L. Friberg; N. Nelson; and V. Vouk. 1978. "Air Pollution and Cancer: Risk Assessment Methodology and Epidemiological Evidence." *Environmental Health Perspectives* 22.

Chiazze, L.; D. Levin; and T. Silverman. 1977. "Recent Changes in Estimated Cancer Mortality." In *Origins of Human Cancer, Book A: Incidence of Cancer in Humans,* edited by H. H. Hiatt, J. D. Watson, and J. A. Winsten. (Cold Spring Harbor Conferences on Cell Proliferation, vol. 4.) New York: Cold Spring Harbor Laboratory.

Cole, P.; and M. B. Goldman. 1975. "Occupation." In *Persons at High Risk of Cancer: An Approach to Cancer Etiology and Control,* edited by J. F. Fraumeni, Jr. New York: Academic Press.

Doernberg, A. 1978. "Energy Use in Japan and the United States." In *International Comparisons of Energy Consumption,* edited by J. Dunkerley. Washington, D.C.: Resources for the Future.

Environmental Protection Agency, Office of Research and Development. 1977. *Air Quality Criteria for Lead.* (EPA-600/8-77-017.) Washington, D.C.: EPA.

————. 1978. "Interim Primary Water Regulations: Control of Organic Chemical Contaminants in Drinking Water." *Federal Register.* 43.

————, Environmental Criteria and Assessment Office, Office of Research and Development. 1979. *Air Quality Criteria for Carbon Monoxide.* Research Triangle Park, N.C.: EPA.

Friberg, L.; M. Piscator; G. Nordberg; and T. Kjellstrom. 1974. *Cadmium in the Environment.* Cleveland, Ohio: CRC Press.

Haenszel, W. 1975. "Migrant Studies." In *Persons at High Risk of Cancer: An Approach to Cancer Etiology and Control,* edited by J. F. Fraumeni, Jr. New York: Academic Press.

Harriss, R. C.; C. Hohenemser; and R. W. Kates. 1978. "Our Hazardous Environment." *Environment* 20.

Higginson, J.; and C. S. Muir. In press. "Environmental Carcinogenesis: Misconceptions and Limitations to Cancer Control." *Journal of the National Cancer Institute.*

Hogstedt, C.; N. Malmqvist; and B. Wadman. 1979. "Leukemia in Workers Exposed to Ethylene Oxide." *Journal of the American Medical Association* 241.

Howe, G. R.; J. D. Burch; A. B. Miller; B. Morrison; P. Gordon; L. Weldon; L. W. Chambers; G. Fodor; and G. M. Winsor. 1977. "Artificial Sweeteners and Human Bladder Cancer." *Lancet* 2.

International Agency for Research on Cancer, Working Group on the Evaluation of the Carcinogenic Risk of Chemicals to Man. 1977. *Asbestos.* (IARC Monographs on the Evaluation of the Carcinogenic Risk of Chemicals to Man, vol. 14.) Lyon, France: IARC.

Jablon, S. 1975. "Radiation." In *Persons at High Risk of Cancer: An Approach to Cancer Etiology and Control,* edited by J. F. Fraumeni, Jr. New York: Academic Press.

Laskin, S.; A. R. Sellakumar; M. Kuschner; N. Nelson; S. La Mendola; G. M. Rusch; G. V. Katz; N. C. Dulak; and R. E. Albert. Forthcoming. "Inhalation Carcinogenicity of Epichlorohydrin."

Levin, D. L.; S. S. Devesa; J. D. Godwin II; and D. T. Silverman. 1974. *Cancer Rates and Risks,* 2d ed. (DHEW Pub. no. [NIH] 76-691.) Washington, D.C.: Government Printing Office.

Linsell, C. A.; and F. G. Peers. 1977. "Aflatoxin and Liver Cell Cancer." *Transactions of the Royal Society of Tropical Medicine and Hygiene* 71.

National Academy of Sciences/National Research Council. 1974. *Air Quality and Automobile Emission Control.* Report by the Coordinating Committee on Air Quality Studies. NAS, Nat. Acad. Eng. vol. 1, Summary Report. Senate Committee on Public Works, U.S. Senate serial no. 93-24. Washington, D.C.: Government Printing Office.

National Cancer Institute, National Institute of Environmental Health Sciences, and National Institute for Occupational Safety and Health. 1978. *Estimates of the Fraction of Cancer in the United States Related to Occupational Factors.* Washington, D.C.: Department of Health, Education and Welfare.

National Institute of Environmental Health Sciences. 1977. *Human Health and the Environment: Some Research Needs.* Report of the Second Task Force for Research Planning in Environmental Health Science to the National Institute of Environmental Health Sciences. (DHEW Pub. no. [NIH] 77-127.) Washington, D.C.: Government Printing Office.

National Institutes of Health/National Cancer Institute, Smoking and Health Program. 1978. *Status Report,* Division of Cancer Cause and Prevention (December).

National Research Council, Safe Drinking Water Committee. 1977. *Drinking Water and Health.* Washington, D.C.: National Academy of Sciences.

———, Committee for a Study of Saccharin and Food Safety Policy. 1978. *Part I, Saccharin and Its Impurities: Technical Assessment of Risks and Benefits* (November). Washington, D.C.: National Academy of Sciences.

Nelson, N. 1976. "The Chloroethers—Occupational Carcinogens: A Summary of Laboratory and Epidemiology Studies." *Annals of the N.Y. Academy of Science* 271.

New York State Department of Health. 1978. *Love Canal—Public Health Time Bomb.* A special report to the governor and legislature. Albany, New York: NYSDH.

Pocchiari, F.; V. Silano; and A. Zampieri. 1979. "Human Health Effects from Accidental Release of Tetrachlorodibenzo-p-dioxin (TCDO) at Seveso, Italy." *Annals of the N.Y. Academy of Science* 320.

President's Biomedical Research Panel. 1976. Appendix A. Washington, D.C.: Government Printing Office.

Preventive Medicine USA, Theory, Practice, and Application of Prevention in Environmental Health Services: Social Determinants of Human Health, Task Force Reports sponsored by the John E. Fogarty International Center for Advanced Study in the Health Sciences. National Institutes of Health and the American College of Preventive Medicine, PRODIST, New York, 1976.

Savage, E. P. 1977. *National Study to Determine Levels of Chlorinated Hydrocarbon Insecticides in Human Milk, and Supplementary Report to the National Milk Study, 1975–76; 1977.* (PB-284-393.) National Technical Information Service.

Shore, R. E.; B. S. Pasternack; E. U. Thiessen; M. Sadow; R. Forbes; and R. E. Albert. 1979. "A Case Study of Hair Dye Use and Breast Cancer." *Journal of the National Cancer Institute* 62.

U.S. Congress. 1969. Joint Committee on Atomic Energy. Testimony of G. Saccomano, "Uranium Miners' Health." In *Radiation Standards for Uranium Mining.* Hearing before the Subcommittee on Research, Development, and Radiation. 91st Cong., 1st sess., March 17 and 18. Washington, D.C.: Government Printing Office.

Weiss, B.; and W. Simon. 1975. "Quantitative Perspectives on the Long-Term Toxicity of Methyl Mercury and Similar Poisons." In *Behavorial Toxicology,* edited by B. Weiss and G. Laties. New York: Plenum Press.

World Health Organization. 1976a. *Mercury.* Published under the joint sponsorship of the United Nations Environment Program and the World Health Organization. (Environmental Health Criteria: 1.) Geneva: World Health Organization.

———. 1976b. *Polychlorinated Biphenyls and Terphenyls.* Published under the joint sponsorship of the United Nations Environmental Program and the World Health Organization. (Environmental Health Criteria: 2.) Geneva: World Health Organization.

ASBESTOS AND UNNECESSARY DEATHS

Irving J. Selikoff, M.D.
Director, Division of Environmental Medicine
Mount Sinai School of Medicine

About 100 years ago we began to understand the causes of disease, with the discovery of various infections such as tuberculosis, streptococcus, and diphtheria. About fifty years ago we began to learn something of metabolic diseases. It must have been a remarkable decade in the 1920s when in a few short years we discovered facts about pernicious anemia, pellegra, and diabetes. Then, as Dr. Nelson pointed out, twenty-five or thirty years ago there began to be increasing awareness of exogenous causes of disease—environmental causes if you like, but I think exogenous is better, since it includes the various cultural or lifestyle factors that have been mentioned. Dr. Nelson also said, with justice, that most of the advances, apart perhaps from replacement therapy, have been made in terms of prevention.

If causes of disease are now different and if we're going to make additional progress, it's likely that the means of prevention will also have to change. I don't think that having more sewers or better pasteurization or cleaner water is going to do this for us. In a sense, there will have to be a new preventive medicine, for it's very difficult to see where this kind of prevention fits into our current medical care system. To the extent that Blue Cross and Blue Shield Plans are part of that medical system, one wonders, if they remain unchanged, whether they will be relevant to the problems we are going to face. Is the prevention going to be for the individual or for the general public?

By and large, Blue Shield and Blue Cross Plans have been focused on the individual, whether in the hospital or the doctor's office, or even in the corporate medical department. But the kind of changes that will be required for the prevention of exogenously induced disease involve large populations and the general public. Are educational programs going to be the responsibility of the National Cancer Institute and HEW, or of the health insurers? It's a fair question.

We've been studying a number of groups of workers exposed to asbestos and a variety of other exogenous agents, ranging from vinyl chloride to polychlorinated biphenyls. In one study we've been following members of the International Association of Heat and Frost Insulators and Asbestos Workers, who insulate the pipes in large buildings. On January 1, 1967, there were 17,800 men in this union. Since 1964 the risk they were exposed to has been known (Selikoff, Ching, and Hammond 1964). To give some sense of what is happening among groups of this sort, in the decade from 1967 to 1977 there were 2,271 deaths among these 17,800 men. Calculating the expected deaths based on their ages in 1967, there should have been only 1,659. Why were there these extra 612 deaths? Some died of scarred lungs (asbestosis), as you would expect, but the major cause of excess deaths was cancer (Table 4–3). Instead of 320 cancer deaths, 995 occurred. Breaking these down by organ site, instead of 106 deaths from cancer of the lung, there were 486—one out of every 5 of these men died of lung cancer. Instead of zero mortality from mesothelioma (which causes about 1 out of 10,000 deaths in the population), there were 175 deaths. Death rates from cancer of the esophagus, stomach, colon, rectum, kidney, oropharynx, and larynx were also excessive.

These young people enter their trade, just as most workers enter factories, construction trades, shipyards, or whatever, when they're about eighteen, nineteen, or twenty, as apprentices. They then invest their lives in their work. They don't die until they're about fifty or fifty-five. When you look at what happens at thirty to thirty-five years from the onset of their work, one-third of all the deaths were due to lung cancer. This has been a disaster. How relevant was our medical care system? Almost every one of these men had Blue Cross and Blue Shield coverage, negotiated by their union and their employer. What difference did it make? In these ten years, there were virtually none who had had any preventive surveillance, or who had been seen regularly by a doctor or had been a beneficiary of our government's organized medical care approach, in terms of what we might have done to prevent what actually did happen.

Table 4–3 Deaths Among 17,800 Asbestos Insulation Workers in the United States and Canada, January 1, 1967–December 31, 1976

Underlying cause of death	Expected[a]	Observed		Ratio o/e	
		(BE)	(DC)	(BE)	(DC)
Total deaths, all causes	1,658.9	2,271	2,271	1.37	1.37
Total cancer, all sites	319.7	995	922	3.11	2.88
Cancer of lung	105.6	486	429	4.60	4.06
Pleural mesothelioma	b	63	25	.....	.....
Peritoneal mesothelioma	b	112	24	.....	.....
Mesothelioma, n.o.s.	b	0	55	.....	.....
Cancer of esophagus	7.1	18	18	2.53	2.53
Cancer of stomach	14.2	22	18	1.54	1.26
Cancer of colon-rectum	38.1	59	58	1.55	1.52
Cancer of larynx	4.7	11	9	2.34	1.91
Cancer of pharynx, buccal	10.1	21	16	2.08	1.59
Cancer of kidney	8.1	19	18	2.36	2.23
All other cancer	131.8	184	252	1.40	1.91
Noninfectious pulmonary diseases, total	59.0	212	188	3.59	3.19
Asbestosis	b	168	78	.....	.....
All other causes	1,280.2	1,064	1,161	0.83	0.91

[a] Expected deaths are based upon white male age-specific U.S. death rates of the U.S. National Center for Health Statistics, 1967–1976.

[b] Rates are not available, but these have been rare causes of death in the general population.

NOTES: Man-years of observation=166,853.

(BE) = Best evidence. Number of deaths categorized after review of best available information (autopsy, surgical, clinical).

(DC) = Number of deaths as recorded from death certificate information only.

Is this a hopeless situation? By no means; it's hopeless only if we don't do anything. In most cancer (except for a few, like benzene leukemia), as in angiosarcoma of the liver following exposure to vinyl chloride, nasal cancer associated with ·nickel smelting, cancer of the lung connected with smoking, or cancer of the vagina as a consequence of the use of DES, for reasons that we don't quite understand there is a long period of *clinical latency*. For these asbestos-exposed workers, we found that there were very few excess deaths of lung cancer before ten years, and lung cancer doesn't reach a peak until after about thirty to thirty-four years (Figure 4–6). In the case of asbestosis, nothing much happens until twenty-five to forty years from onset of work, and death doesn't occur until the age of fifty or sixty. These deaths reach their peak at forty to forty-

Figure 4–6.   Deaths from Lung Cancer Among 17,800 Asbestos Insulation Workers in the United States and Canada, January 1, 1967 –December 31, 1976, Analysis by Duration from Onset of Employment

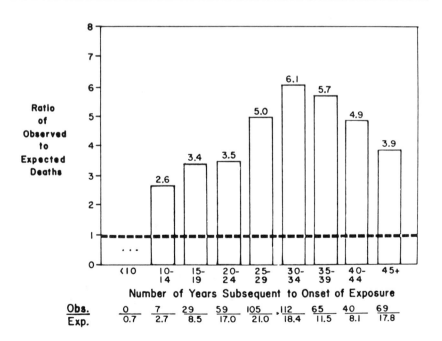

five years from onset (Figure 4–7). Most are totally unnecessary. Scarred lungs are not the cause; that's almost a contradiction. The patients *have* scarred lungs, but they die with superimposed infections, generally inadequately treated. If kept under surveillance by their physicians when infected with bronchitis, bronchopneumonia, or pneumonia, treatment is eminently successful. They may have a rough week or two in the hospital or at home; then they're back on an even keel, with limited activity, but able to continue their lives. Yet many of the 168 such men in this group suffered what might be considered unnecessary deaths because of lack of preventive surveillance and sufficiently timely therapy. Similarly, in mesothelioma, nothing much happens for twenty to twenty-five years; death rates then peak at around forty-five years from onset.

Figure 4–7.   Asbestosis Death Rates Among 17,800 Asbestos Insulation Workers in the United States and Canada, January 1, 1967–December 31, 1976, Analysis by Duration from Onset of Employment

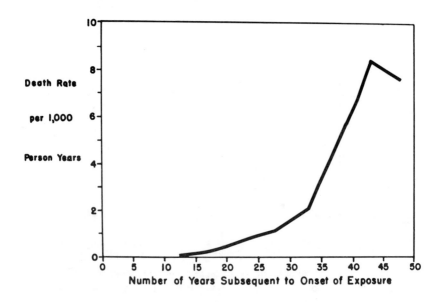

We have a long period in which to intervene, a period of clinical latency, which has not been used, and so this latency, in the past, has been a trap for us, lulling us into a false sense of security until suddenly symptoms appear. We have had virtually no preventive surveillance and have been treating end-stage disease when it's called to our attention. But the latency period also provides an opportunity, because in many cases the course can be reversed. Where it can't be reversed, preclinical diagnosis and therapy provide a challenge for the excellent medical care system that we have developed.

It may be useful to consider the dimensions of the problem. Former HEW Secretary Califano estimated that since World War II there have been somewhere around 8 to 10 million Americans who have been significantly exposed to asbestos at their work. He did not take into account others exposed to it from such consumer products as hair dryers, or even more important, the wives and children who were jeopardized by asbestos dust that these workers brought home from the plants or construction sites on their clothes. In one factory we have been tracing the wives and children who lived with their husbands and fathers in the early 1940s. By last year, among the first 626 we examined, one-third had abnormal x-rays. They felt fine, they were not short of breath, and the asbestosis was minimal in most cases. Yet over 200 of them had asbestosis, with all it forebodes. As we traced these 626, we found five instances of mesothelioma, with one person already dead; they're all dead now. But the point, again, is that not one single group of household contacts has been under preventive surveillance, or has even been examined. Our excellent medical care system has not been used in their behalf for early diagnosis and treatment.

Here is another example, a case that I saw a year ago, a young woman thirty-five years old who was the mother of three children. She suspected she might die because she had mesothelioma (Figure 4–8), and because her dad, who had been a shipyard worker in Quincy, Massachusetts, had died of lung cancer, and her mother of pleural mesothelioma. She had learned a good deal about the condition. She told us that when her dad came home from the shipyard, her mother would shake out his work clothes, and the kids would be playing on the floor nearby. No one in that shipyard, or any of their families, had ever had the advantage of preventive surveillance, despite their good coverage under prepaid medical care insurance.

Figure 4–8.   X-ray of the Lungs of a Woman with Right Pleural Mesothelioma of One Year's Duration. Surgery and chemotherapy proved ineffective; the patient died of tracheal compression by invading tumor.

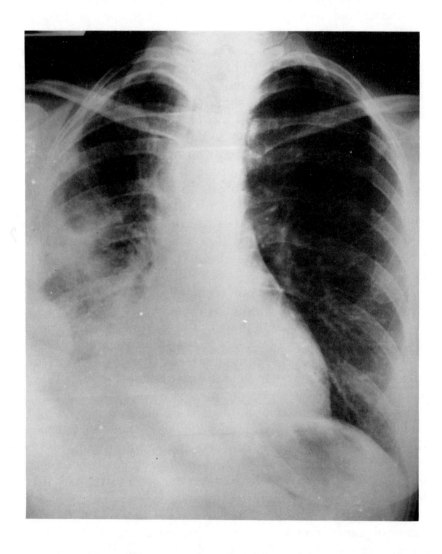

Table 4–4 Age-Standardized Lung Cancer Death Rates for Cigarette Smoking and/or Occupational Exposure to Asbestos Dust

Group	Exposure to Asbestos?	History Cigarette Smoking?	Death Rate	Mortality Difference	Mortality Ratio
Control	No	No	11.3	0.0	1.00
Asbestos workers	Yes	No	58.4	+47.1	5.17
Control	No	Yes	122.6	+111.3	10.85
Asbestos workers	Yes	Yes	601.6	+590.3 ±	53.24

NOTE: Rate per 100,000 man-years standardized for age on the distribution of the man-years of 12,051 asbestos workers followed prospectively 1967–1976. Controls included 73,763 like men in a prospective study at the American Cancer Society for the same decade. Number of lung cancer deaths based on death certificate information.

Dr. Nelson reported on the interaction between various agents, and these conform to our most recent data. When we look among asbestos workers at those who did and did not smoke, using as controls the people in an American Cancer Society study, we found that among those who did not smoke or work with asbestos, the death rate for lung cancer per year was 11 per 100,000. For asbestos workers who didn't smoke it was 58, or five times as much. Smokers who didn't work with asbestos had a rate of 122. When that already very high rate was multiplied by exposure to asbestos, it went up to 601 (Table 4–4). We then found among those who in 1967 had been smoking, one group that had stopped and another that had continued. By 1970 we ascertained that *if an asbestos worker stops smoking, his risk of dying of lung cancer is reduced to one-half or one-third of that of his colleagues who continue to smoke.* If you do nothing else but educate exposed workers about the importance of their special risk from the combination of asbestos and smoking and their special need to stop smoking, you can probably save far more lives than can all the thoracic surgeons and radiotherapists in our country.

Therefore, the question now very much before us is whether we are going to meet the challenge of preventive surveillance. It is not a question of new technology, but of new thinking. Our health care system is based primarily on private individual medical care, one to one, with the best possible therapy for established disease. There are currently no public health mechanisms to turn to for long-term surveillance of large groups. Health insurers have had only limited commitment to preventive surveillance in the past—will this change? That depends upon health insurance and industry leadership; if it doesn't, some other solution, some alternate means, may have to be found. If this facet of disease prevention is not dealt with, we will not utilize the science that Dr. Nelson described to meet the opportunities and challenges that will be with us in the future.

Reference

Selikoff, I.; I. Ching; and E. Hammond. 1964. "Asbestos Exposure and Neoplasia." *Journal of the American Association.*

INDUSTRY AND HEALTH CARE

Richard H. Egdahl, M.D.
Director, Health Policy Institute Boston University

Industry today has two major involvements in health, one in assuring a healthy workplace through accident and disease prevention, and the other in financing—and sometimes providing—health services for employees and their families.

Industry is involved in a very wide range of cost containment, health promotion, and health care delivery programs. Employee health benefits are at the very core of the national health insurance debate—as well as labor-management negotiations—and, indeed, at the heart of whatever restructuring of incentives is developed for patients and providers.

We have been investigating three questions within the general realm of industry and health. First, should corporate medical departments expand their primary-care activities? And if they do, can confidentiality issues be solved? Is the corporate medical director—who is often responsible for Occupational Safety and Health Administration (OSHA) control—also the doctor of the employee, or is he working principally for the corporation? There are some arguments for expanding the availability of primary-care services in corporate settings, and I will touch on those. Second, can workable utilization review programs be developed in the private sector? And, third, can physicians be paid on a fee-for-service basis and function effectively in health maintenance organizations (HMOs) that are offered by a corporation to its employees?

On the corporate primary-care question, we have a model program in Boston. The Gillette Company, based there, offers a very wide range of primary-care services for employees. The "company" physicians also practice in private offices and use the same charts at corporate and private office sites. Complete confidentiality of records exists. These employees, and in many cases their families as well, look on the medical director and his staff as personal physicians. The medical department had 45,000 visits in 1976, of which 43,000 were for complaints classified as "nonoccupational" in origin. The interesting thing is that some crude calculations made by Gillette show that the cost of this care, if delivered outside the company, would have been $1.9 million, whereas the medical department's budget was $700,000. So there were considerable savings from the standpoint of overall corporate finances by having a vigorous primary-care activity. Now, this trend has not been encouraged by organized medicine, and there are reasons for not doing it in some corporations, as in situations where the corporate medical staff is perceived by employees as working mainly for the corporation and not as personal physicians. But there are corporations in this country where primary-care services are expanding, and from the standpoint of the employees, to their advantage.

Many companies are very much involved in health services utilization control. Motorola and Caterpillar, among other big organizations, have contracted with foundations for medical care or with professional standards review organizations for utilization review services. Some of them seem to succeed in decreasing hospital use. The Maricopa Foundation for Medical Care in Arizona reviewed hospitalization in a rigorous fashion, and found that bed days for Motorola patients in the area were a little over 5 per 1,000, compared to 7.1 per 1,000 for a control population that was matched by age and sex. And there are similar examples around the country. We're studying these models with particular attention to differences in the control populations. We predict that a partnership involving various methods of utilization control between insurers and industry will grow very rapidly over the next few years. Although a rapid growth of HMOs may occur in the same period, probably not more than 20 percent of the U.S. population will be covered by HMOs in the next decade, and this points to a need for private-sector approaches to utilization problems in unstructured fee-for-service practice.

Deere and Company, a large midwestern corporation producing farm machinery among other products, has a concentration of employees in a few cities and is catalyzing the development of fee-for-service HMOs there. Can doctors paid on a fee-for-service basis be motivated to participate in cost containment? Deere officials are working closely with local doctor groups and

consultants and are finding that physicians are often cooperative because they see the plan as preserving the individualized
practice setting they and their patients value and as decreasing the need for intensified government regulation, which
many fear presages a drift to a national health service.

I think industry in the 1980s and 1990s will increasingly
develop top-level corporate strategic planning of health-related
activities and will link this planning process to an employee
health information base. In many corporations, the various
health care and health-related programs that now exist are not
coordinated or considered as a unitary system at the level of
executive vice presidents or chief executives. But I believe the
important relationship between dangerous situations—either
accidents or environmental toxins—and health benefit costs
will increasingly be recognized. In addition, cost containment
programs and health promotion activities in many corporations are now almost totally separate in terms of reporting
functions. When one looks at the entire spectrum of activities
that have to do with health, one sees the need for some coordinating force at a high executive level, which currently does not
exist except in a very few corporations.

Over the next twenty years we will see the development of
integrated employee health information bases that will be used
to develop utilization control programs, monitor health promotion programs, assess absenteeism, and evaluate benefits programs. To some extent, this development will necessitate
alterations in current data systems, admittedly a problem.
And yet I see this as one of the cardinal challenges to private
health insurers. The interrelationship of these various health
activities is logical. What justification is there for health promotion activities left uncoordinated with health benefits, or
with OSHA-mandated activities, or with employee assistance
programs, when all involve the health of employees and their
families?

Techniques will have to be developed to solve problems of
confidentiality. In addition, there is a great challenge to clean
up the data, since studies show that many currently obtained
are inaccurate. Nevertheless, there are some careful studies in
which data problems have been overcome; for example, one
done at AT&T that showed that there is less absenteeism in a

group of workers enrolled in an HMO, compared to a control population. Morale and stress factors in the workplace are taking on increased salience, and techniques are being devised, in association with the Rand Insurance Study, for measuring health status in new ways. A fundamental concern of the senior executives in a corporation is productivity. I doubt that it will ever be possible to make an ironclad case for causal connections between available health programs and worker productivity. But I believe it does make sense for management and labor together to strive toward a healthy and happy workplace, which may roughly correlate with efficiency, motivation, and, overall, a more productive company.

I think that industry, working in partnership with insurers and providers, will be *a* major force in determining the future of the health care delivery system, and *the* major force in creating healthy and productive workplaces, which is where the majority of adult Americans spend most of their working hours.

5 SMALL FUTURES, SICK FUTURES, SHORT FUTURES: INEQUITY AND IRRELEVANCE IN U.S. HEALTH CARE STRATEGIES

H. Jack Geiger, M.D.
Professor of Community Medicine, City College of New York

Dr. Jack Geiger currently is the Arthur C. Logan Professor of Community Medicine at the School of Biomedical Education, City College of New York, a six-year medical school devoted to training physicians for primary care in the inner city. Through his development of a new concept of community health, embodying the needs and resources of the population not only for health care but housing, food, income, and welfare services, the lives of millions of people, especially the poor, have been directly affected. His fight to improve total health care, including efforts to provide self-sufficiency and dignity to the populations served, has conveyed his philosophy that the provision of health services can be an instrument to achieve broad social change. Dr. Geiger's community health programs for Mound Bayou, Mississippi, and the Columbia Point area of Boston have been so emulated in other communities that they are now a part of the mainstream of American medical care. Dr. Geiger has served on numerous commissions and committees, including a special advisory committee on health and poverty for the U.S. Department of Health, Education and Welfare. Co-author of The Training of Good Physicians, *Dr. Geiger's leadership in the genesis and development of community health centers is cited in almost every contemporary text on the U.S. health care system.*

It is perhaps distressing, at what is, after all, essentially a celebration of the achievements of the past half-century and an optimistic commitment to progress in the next half-century, to begin with such a bleak title and such an angry stance. It would be more comfortable to review the very considerable achievements of medicine over the past five decades and to join in confident predictions of fresh triumphs in the future. But one of the most important functions of community medicine, I believe, is to maintain the capacity for outrage—outrage at needless suffering and death, determination in tracking down their causes, and passion in combating them—that has always informed medicine as a social enterprise. And that, in turn, requires at the outset that we focus on our failures, confront the problems we have avoided, and face the contradictions we have ignored.

The failure that, in my view, most urgently commands our outrage, our determination, and our passion is at once social and medical. For all the absolute achievements in the improvement of health status in the United States in the past fifty years, we have failed to close the gap between the top and the bottom, between the experience of the richest and the poorest, between the dominant majority and the ethnic minorities.

Fifty, one hundred, two hundred years ago, all the indicators of harm—morbidity, mortality, infant mortality, disability, all the indices of ill health and early death—were firmly associated with poverty and race, and we knew it. The same is still true today. Although the absolute levels of morbidity and mortality have, over that time, declined dramatically for both rich and poor, white and nonwhite, and though the categories of disease have changed for both, the inequality in most indicators of health status is as great, or nearly as great, as ever. It is an endlessly recurring, endlessly maintained, endlessly unsolved gap. It is hardly necessary to document that gap in detail. A few examples will suffice:

1. Overall U.S. mortality rates began an accelerated decline in the 1970s after twenty years of only modest gains. Yet the overall mortality of racial minorities is still one-third greater than that of whites, and higher rates are also observed among the poor and less educated.

2. The chance of death in the first year and every subsequent year of early life are much higher for poor children, and highest of all for poor black children. While significant improvements in infant mortality have occurred among both whites and racial minorities, the nonwhite rate of decrease was lower until only recently. Racial minorities have almost twice the infant mortality of whites, and the frequency of almost all known risk factors remains higher in the nonwhite population.

3. The gap in longevity has narrowed only slightly. The predicted life expectancy at birth for racial minorities in 1975 was over five years shorter than that of whites.

4. Nonwhites have over three times the maternal mortality of whites, and this differential has not been reduced significantly in the past twenty-five years.

5. In 1975, the age-adjusted death rate among the disadvantaged was higher for four of the five leading causes of death. Although the differential has decreased slightly, in 1975 the white age-adjusted death rate from heart disease was 217.2 per 100,000, compared to 245.2 for all other races.

6. From 1950 to 1975, the age-adjusted cancer death rate for the total U.S. population increased 4 percent. For the white population, the increase was 3 percent during this period; for nonwhites, the increase was 20 percent.

7. The prevalence of poor health, poor nutrition, and slower physical development among children is greater as income decreases. In probable association with nutritional factors, poverty is also strongly associated with mental retardation; some 90 percent of children labeled marginally retarded come from poor families, but have no known organic brain damage.

8. Local studies of children in poverty are the most compelling. In a low-income Chicano community in Los Angeles, children are found to have four times as much amebic dysentery as the national average, twice as much measles, mumps, and tuberculosis, and 1.4 times as much hepatitis. In Nashville, the Meharry study of 1,266 poor families showed that 97 percent of the children had serious health problems. In 1976, the Children's Defense Fund estimated

that 300 to 400 poor children die annually of lead poisoning, and that 6,000 a year suffer lead-induced brain damage.

These appalling social and medical facts are known, and long have been known, to health workers and the general public alike. Periodically—indeed, cyclically—we rediscover them, focus on them, and respond to them. Our responses are almost unvarying: We work to enlarge the provision of medical care services to individuals, we struggle toward universal entitlement to medical care and toward sharp and differential increases in medical care utilization by the poor and nonwhite. We do so for a variety of reasons: a commitment to equality of access to the medical care system; a belief in the right to have care on the basis of need, without limitation by income, social status, or race; and an apparent conviction that medical care to individuals will ultimately change the health status of populations. On the public health side, we have emphasized individual preventive services, called for changes in individual lifestyles and behaviors, and targeted programs to limit the effects, but only rarely to remove the causes, of hazards in the biological and physical environments.

The evidence is overwhelming, I believe, that such responses—unaccompanied by other strategies, other changes—fail. They have not reduced, and cannot reduce, the health status gap. Further, they reflect a deep conceptual and philosophical error in the analysis of the relationship between social circumstance and health status. They represent a way of avoiding other commitments, particularly to structural change in some of the basic patterns of our society, including its mechanisms for the distribution of income, opportunity, power, and experience. By focusing on equality of access to, and utilization of, medical care services rather than on changes and interventions likelier to produce equality of health status, they are, at the least, irrelevant and, at the worst, a method of preserving inequity.

A paradigm for these drastic conclusions is offered by a very recent major study of a different but basic kind of social intervention, that of education, conducted for the Carnegie Council on Children by Richard H. deLone: "Small Futures: Children,

Inequality, and the Limits of Liberal Reform." (1979) Its parallels to our struggles and our failures in health care are so compelling that it is worth attempting to summarize it briefly here.

The study attempts to demonstrate that equal opportunity in America—a tenet central to our liberal ideology—is a myth; that children born into poverty (over one-quarter of every generation) have slim chances of rising out of that poverty; and that, despite decades of liberal reform programs, from the Jacksonian era through the Great Society, the odds against upward mobility for the poor have scarcely changed since the nineteenth century.

The stimulus to reform, deLone argues, has always been the evidence of visible extremes of inequality. Our American uneasiness is over the persistence of profound relative poverty in the midst of relative affluence even in the absence of an American impulse toward radical leveling and complete equality of condition. In the effort to ameliorate inequality, he says, liberal reformers have always had a choice of two different strategies. One is to make profound direct changes in the distribution of wealth and privilege in the society—to alter the ground rules, the focus of decisionmaking, the means of decisionmaking, and the nature of decisions in both the economic and political spheres. The second is to avoid such fundamental structural change and concentrate instead on assistance to individuals. Liberal reformers have consistently chosen the latter.

In education, deLone continues, children have had to carry the burden of change. Liberal reformers encouraged Americans to "defer the dream" for a generation, assuming that children, given a fair shake through individual education, would be upwardly mobile. Rather than trying to modify directly the distribution of economic rewards and special standings, we have concentrated on uplifting the next generation. For well over a century, Americans have believed that a crucial way to make our society more just was by improving our children.

"Confronted with unacceptable economic and social inequalities," the study notes, "we have reflexly channeled our moral indignation into efforts to improve the morality, character, skills, and intelligence of children—especially those who are poor, immigrant, or nonwhite—trusting that by so doing we would reduce social, economic, and racial inequality in the next generation ...

"But in the end, such reforms have failed ... because they were not accompanied by more direct and structural change. Without structural change, education and efforts to equalize opportunity can at best only change the cast of characters who occupy preexisting numbers of positions on the top and on the bottom. The distance between top and bottom and the size of each group—in short, the inequalities that spurred reform in the first place—simply cannot be altered by education" (1979).

The evidence of the failure of reform strategy is in the *current* "arithmetic of inequality" in America. Given two second-graders *of equal ability and test performance,* one from a family in the top 10 percent of U.S. income distribution and the other from a family in the bottom 10 percent, the richer child is four times as likely to enter college, twelve times as likely to complete it, and twenty-seven times as likely, with an average of four more years of schooling than the poorer child, to land a job that will ultimately pay him an income in the top tenth of all incomes. The poorer child has only about one chance in eight of earning even a *median* income.

When it becomes evident that reform through individual assistance has failed, the study argues, it is rarely considered that instead of trying to reduce inequality by helping individuals, we may be able to help individuals by reducing inequality, by recognizing that the dynamics of our social structure are not likely to produce more equality of opportunity unless there is more equality to begin with. Instead, "when individuals fail to profit from the 'help' they receive, the blame may be laid on the individual ... Blaming the victim ... has been a pervasive habit in the history of liberal reform." At its most vicious, it appears as a form of racism, proclaiming that the poor—especially minorities, who are disproportionately poor—are genetically debased. Indeed, resurrection of the genetic hypothesis is often the final stage of reform. As the cycle completes itself, liberalism's emphasis on the individual serves equally well as the rallying cry for racism, individual blame, and reaction.

In a sense, deLone concludes, "Liberalism's focus on.the individual has resulted in a betrayal of liberalism's concern for the individual. By ignoring or dismissing the extent to which social class, social dynamics, and institutional structures affect individuals and their options, social policy has implicitly stacked the deck against some individuals, consigning them to small futures from childhood onward."

In health care, similarly, we have, over and over again, chosen the strategy of individual assistance rather than structural social change. We have opted only, or primarily, for increased access to individual medical care services, despite the evidence of a dozen studies that increased utilization of such services (and the poor in the United States are now equal consumers of medical care, at or above the median) does not rapidly or significantly alter the health status of poor populations. In public health and medical care alike we have focused on individual behaviors and lifestyles, studiously ignoring the context—the social, economic, and environmental determinants of those lifestyles—let alone the large issue of the extent to which social, economic, and political structures impinge on health and block preventive efforts.

Medical care itself, and the education that trains professionals for it, are organized and oriented toward the individual. We struggle to reduce the blood pressure in an individual hypertensive man or woman, to increase the hemoglobin in a single anemic child. We do not, as physicians, usually define our responsibility as attempting to alter the blood pressure or hemoglobin distributions in a defined population, nor are we well organized to do so; and if such efforts are made, in a public health sector, they are usually quite separate from the day-to-day entrepreneurial practice of medicine.

Let me, then, rewrite deLone in terms of health problems: Without structural change, medical care and efforts to equalize opportunity for good health status can only change the cast of characters who occupy preexisting numbers of positions on the top and on the bottom. The distance between the top and the bottom and the size of each group—in short, the inequalities that spurred reform in the first place—simply cannot be altered by medical care alone.

And again: Health care's focus on the individual has resulted in a betrayal of health care's concern for the individual. By
ignoring or dismissing the extent to which social class, social
dynamics, and institutional structures affect individuals and
their health options, health strategy has implicitly stacked the
deck against some individuals, consigning them to small futures, sick futures, short futures.

In education, the deLone study argues, the persistent choice
of individual rather than structural or income-redistributing
strategies stems from our inability to resolve some of the contradictions between economic liberalism and political liberalism—a free-market model producing large and inegalitarian
disparities in wealth as incentives for effort, rewards for enterprise, and spurs for mobility on the one hand, and a political
model committed to the greatest possible equality on the other.
It may be that health strategy is even more vulnerable to the
tensions between a capitalist economy and a democratic polity,
for medical care itself is a major industry, faithfully reflecting
the larger entrepreneurial political economy in its efforts to
maximize income and preserve its autonomy. In consequence,
the medical care establishment has, in the last decade, moved
slowly, but ever more strongly, toward support of universal entitlement and some form of national health insurance, increasing its income while opposing or ignoring structural change.

Now, these are hardly new charges against the predominant
medical care institutions and the health strategies they foster,
and the defensive arguments against these charges are familiar to all of us: that it is neither the province nor the expertise
of medicine to intervene in social policy and that the public
has given medicine no mandate for such efforts, but rather demands of us good, effective, and technically sophisticated curative medicine. And that curative medicine is demonstrably a
good and successful thing, that its failures and defects are determined by socioeconomic problems, not medical ones, and
that our progress is dramatic and is accelerating. It's not our
fault that, no matter how fast the locomotive goes, the caboose
never catches up; something must be wrong with those people!

Yet an outraged and passionate argument for medicine's involvement in social change has been around for a long time. In

1854—125 years ago—John Simon, a physician and the first health officer of the City of London, wrote:

> I would beg any educated person to consider what are the conditions in which alone life can thrive; to learn, by personal inspection, how far those conditions are realized for the masses of our population; and to form for himself a conscientious judgment as to the need for great, even revolutionary, reforms. Let any such person devote an hour to visiting some very poor neighborhood in the metropolis . . . let him breathe its air, taste its water, eat its bread. Let him think of human life struggling there for years . . . Let him gravely reflect whether such sickening evils . . . ought to be the habit of our laboring population: whether the legislature, which his voice helps to constitute, is doing all that might be done to palliate these wrongs; whether it be not a jarring discord in the civilization we boast, that such things continue, in the midst of us, scandalously neglected. . . .
>
> If there be citizens so destitute that they can afford to live only where they must straightaway die—renting the twentieth straw-heap in some lightless feverbin, or breathing from the cesspool and the sewer; so destitute that they can buy no water—that milk and bread must be impoverished to meet their means of purchase— that the drugs sold them for sickness must be rubbish or poison; surely no civilized community dare avert itself from the care of this abject orphanage. . . If such conditions of food or dwelling are absolutely inconsistent with healthy life, what more final test of poverty can there be, or what clearer right to public succour, than that the subject's means fall short of providing him other conditions than these? (1870)

The central contribution of community medicine in the United States over the last several decades, I believe, is that it has accepted John Simon's challenge: That is, it has worked simultaneously for individual assistance through increased access to medical care *and* for direct intervention of health care programs in efforts toward structural change in the society. There is no a priori reason, after all, why we cannot try to run the equation backwards: If social, economic, and political inequities are major contributors to inequality in health status, then why can't we design medical care institutions and health care programs to attempt, in addition to their more conventional tasks, social, economic, and political change?

At the peak of the most recent cyclic wave of reform, in the mid-1960s, the invention—or reinvention, or transformation— of neighborhood health centers and their funding as a major effort of the Office of Economic Opportunity provided an opportunity for such attempts at a number of settings—not only in rural Mississippi, where my colleagues and I worked, but in South Carolina, Boston, Chicago, the South Bronx, and Los Angeles. In the face of appalling poverty, inequity, racism, and preventable illness and death, health workers at these and other sites did what made sense. In addition to providing medical care to defined communities, with responsibility for improvement in the health status of both individuals and populations, they attempted to organize those communities and to help them become politically active and effective in their own health and health-related interests. Voting rights and political action led, in turn, to some redistribution of income and employment opportunities, to some redistribution of relevant governmental services, and to greater control over hazards in the environment. Where hunger was widespread and there were no other remedial resources, medical care funds paid for meat and milk and vegetables; literally filling "prescriptions" for these and similar necessities followed quite naturally from the observation that the specific therapy for malnutrition is food. Where abysmal housing was linked directly to infection, trauma, and exposure to toxins, medical care funds (and community organization) accomplished repair and construction. Where unemployment and lack of education blocked upward mobility—and the frequent concomitant improvement in health status—medical care funds paid for jobs and training, and in a few instances helped to launch self-sustaining enterprises in fields other than medical care.

Those days are gone—killed by the society's resistance to redistribution, by the charges of excessive costs (since the so-called "externalities" of increased potential, increased productivity, increased quality of life, and increased years of life did not appear on the account books of any institution), and by the victim-blaming that characterizes troughs in the reformist cycle. An important residue of principle remains, however, and it has affected much of our thinking about health care. It is clearer, now, that individual medical care need not be separated from public health, that the two can be combined under one roof in programs responsive and accountable to defined and coherent populations or communities, even in private-sector models of care. Intervention in the workplace is a surviving—and growing—form of medical care concern over the environment. The right of consumers to have a determining say in the organization and provision of health services is established in law, if not yet in practice. A growing number of health status deficiencies are recognized as political and economic rather than merely technical issues, as wounds not only in individual bodies but in the body politic.

I have called these principles a residue. They are, simultaneously, an *agenda* for community medicine in the next fifty years. Recognition of the ineffectiveness of individual medical care in changing the health status of populations, in closing the health gap, is not an argument against universal entitlement to such services, which is eminently justifiable on grounds of equity and the quality of life. It is, rather, an argument for its combination with efforts to accomplish income redistribution, family services, full employment, and some reallocation of power and decisionmaking. Medicine has a stake in these issues and a role to play in their resolution. Community medicine has the task of finding the new organizational forms, conducting the experiments, and maintaining the outrage, the passion, and the commitment that may lead to wiser and more effective strategy choices when the reformist cycle peaks again.

References

deLone, R. and Carnegie Council on Children. 1979. *Small Futures: Inequality and the Limits of Liberal Reform*. New York: Harcourt Brace Jovanovich.

Simon, J. 1870. "A Ministry of Health," May 15, 1854, in City of London Reports. London: Eyre and Spottswood, Her Majesty's Printers.

THE NEED FOR STRUCTURAL CHANGE

Victor W. Sidel, M.D.
Chairman, Department of Social Medicine
Montefiore Hospital Medical Center

Not infrequently medical students or house officers from one of the two medical schools in New York in which I teach—the School for Biomedical Education at City College and the Albert Einstein College of Medicine—or from other schools, come to me in despair: "What is this profession that I've gotten into? In coming to medical school I imagined an opportunity to truly be of help to people, to help change some of the conditions that lead to sickness rather than simply learning how to put Band-Aids on the wounds." My response is to tell them of Jack Geiger's work. I tell them that not all doctors share the narrow and self-serving views they have encountered. I tell them there are indeed some doctors—an increasing number—who view medicine as more than an opportunity to "do well by doing good," to demonstrate technical virtuosity, and to gain satisfaction and power from the needs and dependence of patients. These doctors, I say, see medicine as an opportunity to identify and help change some of the conditions that lead to ill health, to participate in strengthening the autonomy and the power of patients and their communities, and to help reorganize a technologically muscle-bound, tunnel-visioned, anachronistic, and profit-and-power-oriented medical care system. One role model I offer them—of someone who has consistently and effectively developed these functions over the past twenty years—is Jack Geiger.[a]

I want to add here some specific examples of the problems he discusses, and especially to provide a glimpse of the Bronx, and of the needs that health workers must respond to. Another objective is to suggest some responses, from other countries and from our own.

[a] The two decades of his work are spanned, for example, in Geiger (1957, 1976).

How one looks at the problems of health and illness depends almost entirely on the community one is looking at and its social and economic circumstances. Professor Fein asked us to examine the possibility that as energy supplies become tighter, as there is a slowdown in the economy, and, for these and other reasons, as resources become less available, there will be diminished willingness of those who have much to permit the levels of taxation that can provide adequate human services for those who have little. These public services, he reminds us, are based largely on the wealth of an expanding economy, so that no one has to give up any current standard of living—only to sacrifice a small part of the annual increase in that standard—to help others. To this problem of diminished growth must be added the ravages of inflation on those with small or fixed incomes and the ravages of a shift in public expenditures from human services to armaments. When these occur, those who are poorest, and therefore weakest, in our society will be the ones from whom resources are most withdrawn. My message is that this scenario is already unfolding. Mine is not the view south from the playing fields of Yale or west from the Court of St. James. My view is east from Yankee Stadium into the South Bronx, into one of the highest, if not the highest, concentrations of poverty and disease in any affluent country in the world. It is an area with one of the worst records for residential fires seen anywhere in the world, fires born of social and economic conditions, whose end result—the end-stage of this particular disease—is vast areas of rubble that look like London after the blitz. President Carter stood on Charlotte Street looking at this scene and promised to help, but of course has not.

When it comes to occupational health and safety, here is a picture of a small dress factory in the South Bronx (Figure 5-1). The working conditions in that building are unspeakable in any society and are obscene in a rich one. Yet "honorable men" at this moment are trying to tear down the limited protection that the Occupational Safety and Health Administration offers in small factories like this in the United States.

It is almost impossible to tell you how many people live in the South Bronx, because the U.S. census undercounts people living in such areas. Many of them are undocumented and un-

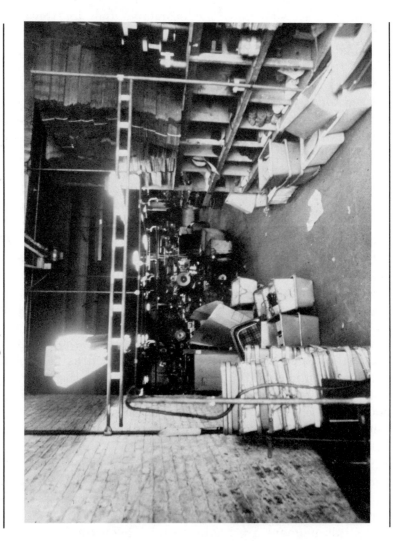

Figure 5-1   Photograph of Small Dress Factory in South Bronx

counted persons, people whom we call "illegal aliens" even as we encourage their entrance into the United States to do the jobs no one else wants to do at pay scales no one else will accept. At the least, there are 500,000 people living in this kind of environment in the Bronx alone. In New York City alone there are probably some 2 million people growing up and living under these kinds of conditions—some 1 percent of the population of the United States, just within one city. Overall in the United States we are probably talking about somewhat less than Franklin Delano Roosevelt's "one-third of a nation."

Meanwhile, a few blocks away from these scenes, a distance one can cover on high-speed highways in less than five minutes, there are scenes of enormous wealth in the Northwest Bronx. The change in health conditions and in health statistics that those five minutes represent is staggering. Tables 5–1 and 5–2 show some of the differences between Health Planning District A in the South Bronx and District E a few blocks away in the North Bronx.

Leaving the question of preventive medicine aside for the moment and thinking just of medical care, it is my opinion—and I know it is a controversial one—that in a rational and humane society, the people in those areas that have the greatest needs for medical care should have the greatest access to medical care services. In fact, as we are all aware, in most places in the United States the correlation is in the opposite direction. Thus, Morrisania City Hospital in the South Bronx was closed three years ago; the Fordham Hospital, located at the top end of the South Bronx, is now a parking lot. These two hospitals have been replaced; indeed they have been replaced by a $100-million facility. But the location of that facility is not the South Bronx, but the North Bronx. This decision was a careful and rational one, based on the finest principles of health planning, with attention to questions of economies of scale, of regionalization, of professional education, and of technical quality of medical care. But the net result was the removal of additional jobs from the South Bronx, of community stability, and of the modicum of power that comes from having powerful institutions in the neighborhood. In short, the medical care system, which overall constitutes almost 10 percent of

Table 5-1 Disease and Death Rates for Two Health Districts of Bronx, New York, and for New York City, 1970 (Per 100,000 Population)

	Reported Incidence			Cause of Death		
	Gonorrhea	Lead Poisoning	Measles	Tuberculosis	Accidents	Drug Dependence
Bronx health district A	674	67	30	61	28	24
Bronx health district E	69	2	2	10	32	1
New York City	432	34	15	33	23	9

SOURCE: Comprehensive Health Planning Agency for the City of New York. *Health Planning District Profiles*, CHPA-NYC, profiles for District A and District E in the Bronx, New York.

Table 5–2   Infant Health Indicators for Two Health Districts of Bronx, New York, and for New York City, 1975

	Infant Mortality[a]	Neonatal Mortality[a]	Postneonatal Mortality[a]	Percent Inadequate Prenatal Care
Bronx health District A	23.6	17.7	5.9	31.9
Bronx health District E	9.3	6.9	2.4	14.9
New York City	17.9	13.5	4.7	16.3

SOURCE: Health Systems Agency of New York City. 1978. *Health Systems Plan 1978*, p. 90. New York.
[a] per 1,000 live births.

the GNP and 7 percent of the employment in our society, takes the economic and social support that it can give to these kinds of areas and, for possibly valid technical reasons (at least in the short term), moves them to more affluent areas.

We're not just talking about inpatient services. Even where there was ambulatory care in the South Bronx, the resources are being withdrawn. Almost no physicians live, or have private offices, in the area. There are some shared health facilities, the "Medicaid mills," with patients "Ping-Ponged" from doctor to doctor in attempts to magnify the ridiculously low (in comparison to the medical care needs) Medicaid reimbursement rate, with facilities locked up at night, usually with little attempt at continuity or comprehensiveness of care and almost no preventive medicine. Publicly operated ambulatory care facilities are being decimated.

Finally, large numbers of the people in this area are from Hispanic America. Their culture and their language—and the lack of respect they find in the "mainstream" medical care facilities—lead them to seek help from *botanicas, espiritistas, santeros,* drug shops, and indigenous health aides, and a whole panoply of alternative forms of care. (An excellent recent review of Hispanic folk healers in urban America can be found in Delgado [1979].) For many medical problems such care may be efficient and effective but, since it has essentially no communication with the other form of medical care, patients fall between the cracks, are torn between the two systems of medicine, and may end up losing the benefits of both.

These problems are, of course, not limited to the South Bronx and are not all of recent origin. Data showing two measures of health care needs (restricted-activity days and bed-disability days) and relative number of physician visits (for diagnosis and treatment and for preventive care) by family income are shown in Figures 5–2 and 5–3. It is clear, from these and other measures, that the health care needs of a group increase sharply with decreasing income. It is also clear that, although the number of physician visits for diagnosis and treatment is now roughly equal across income groups, meeting the needs for treatment services would almost certainly require considerably higher accessibility and use by poor people; it is even clearer that preventive services are inequitably distributed. Consequences of this inequity are shown in Figure 5–4 and Tables 5–3 and 5–4. The first two show how the inequitable initial distribution of poliomyelitis immunization in the mid-1950s in some cities of the United States led to a shift in the pattern of subsequent epidemics toward a *greater* burden on poor or black people. This pattern persists, as demonstrated by the data for a diphtheria outbreak in San Antonio in 1970.

The point I'm trying to make, in specific illustrations of Professor Fein's scenario and Dr. Geiger's concerns, is that the scenario and the concerns are not only for the future. The problem exists today and in some ways is getting worse. How shall we—in a society that calls itself "democratic," "just," and "humane"—respond?

There is no question that many of the responses to these problems lie in spheres outside traditional medical concerns, and that some of the relevant models and statistics from other societies are flawed. But there is also no question in my mind that we must look to some of these models and statistics for clues on how to solve some of our problems. There are some definitional and counting differences that muddy transnational comparisons of infant mortality, but these technical differences are small compared to the vast gap between levels of infant mortality for some groups in the United States and those in other countries. And if one looks at infant mortality for babies of poor people and black people compared to others *within* the United States, where the technical differences are minimal, these data can't be swept under the rug, can't be sanitized or expunged. The differences are real and shameful. Furthermore, if one looks at maternal mortality (Table 5–5), or at age-specific mortality for years other than infancy, many industrialized societies do better than we do. To be sure, there are differences in social conditions and in other risk factors, but one cannot help noting that countries of comparable affluence that organize their health services better than we do, do better than we do.

Sweden is a small country and its population is largely homogenous. But Sweden's level of industrialization and per capita gross national product are comparable to those in the United States. As Professor Odin Anderson and others have

Figure 5-2. Relative Number of Physician Visits of Persons with Limited Activity, and of Bed Disability Days, by Family Income (U.S.A., Civilian Non-institutionalized Population, 1975).[1]

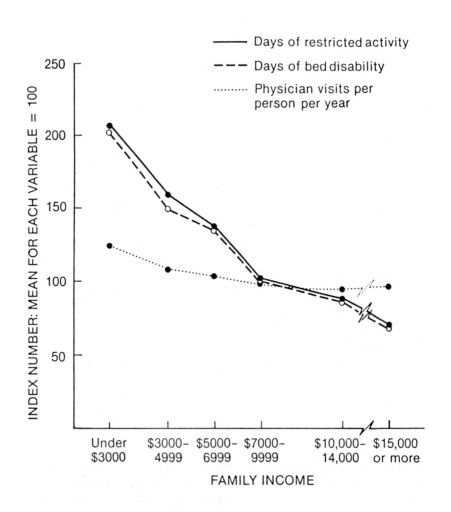

1. Excludes visits to patients in hospitals.

SOURCE: Reprinted with permission from *Medical Care Chartbook*, Seventh Edition, Avedis Donabedian, Solomon J. Axelrod, Leon Wyszewianski, eds. (Ann Arbor: Health Administration Press, 1980), 42 (48).

Figure 5−3. Relative Number of Physician Visits per Person per Year, by Income and Type of Visits (U.S.A., Civilian Non-institutionalized Population, 1975).

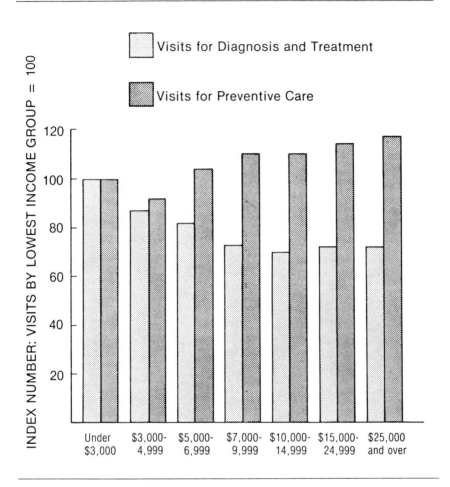

NOTE: Preventive Care visits consists of the following: (a) pre- and post-natal care; (b) routine checkups and checkups for specific purposes such as employment or insurance, in which no diagnosis is made; (c) immunizations provided by a physician or under a physicians's supervision; and (d) visits for eye refractions, for preventive services not included in the preceding categories, and visits for which the type of service provided is unknown.

SOURCE: Reprinted with permission from *Medical Care Chartbook*, Seventh Edition, Avedis Donabedian, Solomon J. Axelrod, Leon Wyszewianski, eds. (Ann Arbor: Health Administration Press, 1980), 42 (48).

Figure 5–4. Distribution of Reported Poliomyelitis Cases, by Census Tract, Kansas City, Missouri, Epidemic years 1946, 1952, and 1959

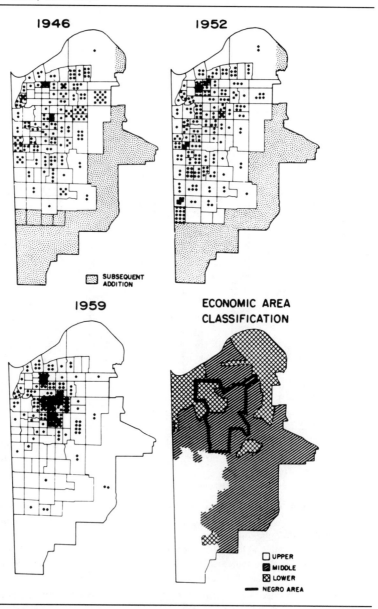

SOURCE: Chin, T. D. Y., and W. M. Marine. 1961. "The Changing Pattern of Poliomyelitis Observed in Two Urban Epidemics." *Public Health Reports* 76, no. 7 (July): 553 –63.

Table 5–3   Poliomyelitis in Des Moines, Iowa

Race and Socioeconomic Group	1952		1959	
	No. of Cases	Cases per 100,000 Population	No. of Cases	Cases per 100,000 Population
White				
Upper	134	224.4	10	15.6
Middle	128	143.3	50	51.5
Lower	50	159.7	42	132.9
Black	3	30.9	33	320.4

SOURCE: Chin, T. D. Y., and W. M. Marine. 1961. "The Changing Pattern of Poliomyelitis Observed in Two Urban Epidemics." *Public Health Reports* 76, no. 7 (July): 553–63.

Table 5–4   Diphtheria Rates in San Antonio, Texas, 1970

	No. of Cases	Cases per 100,000 Population
Ethnic Group		
White—Spanish surname (Chicano)	156	48.6
Black—All surnames	25	45.6
White—non-Spanish surname	15	3.8
Socioeconomic status		
Upper 25%	9	5.6
Middle 50%	78	25.2
Lower 25%	107	62.9

SOURCE: Marcus, E. K., and M. G. Grant. 1973. "Epidemiology of Diphtheria in San Antonio, Texas, 1970." *Journal of the American Medical Association* 224, no. 3 (April): 305–10.

Table 5–5   Maternal Mortality Rates in Selected Countries, 1960–1971 (Deaths Due to Childbirth per 100,000 Live Births)

1960		1971			Percent Decrease 1960—1971
Australia	52.5	Australia	18.5		65
Belgium	40.7	Belgium	20.4	(1970)	50
Canada	44.9	Canada	18.3		59
Denmark	30.2	Denmark	5.3		82
England and Wales	39.5	England and Wales	16.9		57
Finland	71.8	Finland	8.1		89
Japan	130.6	Japan	45.2		65
Netherlands	39.4	Netherlands	12.1		69
Norway	42.0	Norway	19.6		53
Sweden	37.2	Sweden	7.9		79
Switzerland	57.2	Switzerland	27.0		53
U.S.A.	37.1	U.S.A.	20.5		45

SOURCE: Sidel, V. W., and R. Sidel. 1978. *A Healthy State: An International Perspective on the Crisis in United States Medical Care.* New York: Pantheon Books. Derived from Maxwell, R., 1975, *Health Care: The Growing Dilemma,* Table 5, New York, using data drawn from *World Health Statistics Reports,* published regulary by the World Health Organization, Geneva.

described, Sweden has managed to regionalize its health services and organize them on a community basis. District doctors and district nurses are placed in urban neighborhoods, small towns, and rural areas. Pregnant women are provided with good care, beginning in the first trimester and continuing intensively throughout the pregnancy. And these health care services are integrated with appropriate social services. The United States is not poorer than Sweden. We are simply less willing to use our resources to protect the health of all our people.

Great Britain is a country considerably poorer than we are. Its per capita GNP is approximately one-half that of the United States. Furthermore, Great Britain spends only 5.5 percent of its GNP on health care, compared to our 9 percent. In other words, we spend almost $1,000 per person on health care; Great Britain spends almost $350 per person on health care, or one-third as much. Yet in this relatively poor society, the National Health Service has organized and financed health services in such a way that preventive services and primary-care services are preserved and widely accessible, from the posh neighborhoods of London to the mining valleys of Wales. It is true that if one needs certain types of elective surgery one may have to wait a long while. But if I were a child of a poor family or a home-bound older person, I would far rather take my chances with medical care in Great Britain than in the United States.

Very different ideas for dealing with health problems may be found in China, a much poorer country technologically. But China has managed, by a series of integrated methods based on a social and economic revolution, to provide accessible and humane care for its people. All services, including health services, are decentralized locally to the most local level at which those services can be given. Community health workers are selected by, and trained to work with, their neighbors in the preservation and promotion of health. As one example of urban health work, the four women on the right side of Figure 5–5, wearing white hats, are the health workers for their "residents committee" area. This picture was taken during our visit to Xian, a midwestern city, in 1972. The sign over their heads reads "Serve the People," and it was clear that, with limited technology, they served their neighbors well in the areas of preventive medicine and primary care. When we went back to this same health station five years later, the health workers had white coats. They had attained a higher level of technology and training. But because of the social organization of health care, the new technology—at least up to 1977—had been tailored to fit a model for decentralized, accessible, power-diffusing service, rather than service distorted to fit the Procrustean bed of the new technology.

In addition, China has made attempts to integrate its traditional Chinese medicine with what is called "Western medicine." The doctor trained in traditional Chinese methods and the doctor trained in our style of medicine see patients togeth-

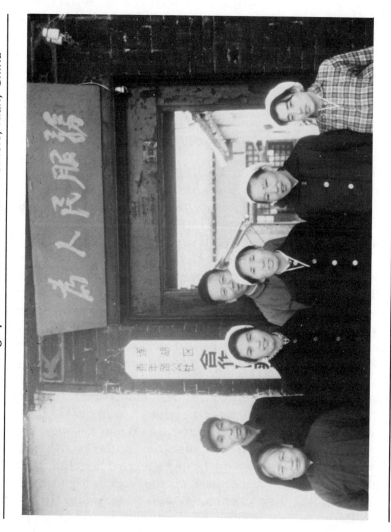

Figure 5–5 Photograph of Chinese Health Workers, Xian, China

er in the clinics. We were told that because of the integration of Western and Chinese medicine, the two doctors are now equivalent in their status. "That sounds fine," we said, "but what would happen if there were a disagreement between them on the advice to be given to the patient?" The response was, to explain the process: Each of the doctors gives his advice to the patient. "If their advice is contradictory," we were told, "it is of course up to the patient to decide whether he will take the advice of the doctor trained in traditional medicine or the doctor trained in Western medicine."

The more interesting issue to me is not the answer. It is the question. Where does the question come from? An advertisement in a U.S. medical journal shows an elderly woman and suggests that "if she could choose her therapy she'd probably choose————." Why can't she choose her therapy, once she has been properly informed of her choices? Another advertisement shows two tablets—one brand name and one generic—and says, "Your patients may not know the difference, but you do." Why *can't* the patient be informed of the possible differences so he can make the choice? The point I want to make is that one of the barriers to the kind of community health service we're talking about is the medical profession itself, a profession that is largely selected, trained, organized, and nurtured in ways that are contrary to people making their own decisions and having control over their own health care.

Can it be done differently? One way we are attempting to implement some of these lessons in the Bronx is in the area surrounding Montefiore Hospital, a lower-middle-class neighborhood where the Department of Social Medicine is training local residents in techniques of health promotion and health prevention in order to help their neighbors. Since they can't be called "barefoot doctors," the name they have chosen for themselves is "health coordinators." One recent event will, I think, give some insight into what Dr. Geiger was talking about when he called for combining medicine with redistribution of power and maintenance of passion and commitment. Because the neighborhood is changing—there are many people now who speak Spanish as their first or only language—the most recent group of health coordinators has had their training entirely in the Spanish language. One of those health coordinators, a thirty-eight-year-old woman from Puerto Rico, was recently involved in a fatal accident. When her family prepared her body for viewing and burial, they clothed her in the dress that she had worn to the graduation from the Community Health Participation Program, wearing the badge that identified her as a "health coordinator." The family told us that this woman had never before in her life graduated from anything. Because she was so proud of learning the skills that permitted her to help her neighbors, to feel more useful, and to be a part of the health of her community, her family felt she would want to be buried with the symbols of her new role. A slogan of the Mothers' Club of the Hispanic group of health coordinators is, "To accomplish great things we must not only act but also dream, not only plan but also believe." It is this capacity for belief in the future and for action now, a capacity medicine today largely takes away from people, that it must give back to them. (For a further development of this theme, see Sidel [1979].)

What is recognized in China and in many other countries, but is still fighting for recognition in the United States, is that health is in large part determined by the ways in which society is organized and the ways in which its services are provided. It is my view that if we are serious about providing better health care and better health for all our people, if we want our nation to be a decent place to live for any of our people, we must begin to deal with medicine not as an entrepreneurial enterprise but as part of a social service. We must begin to use medicine, with its huge budgets, its enormous employment, and its ability to distribute resources for either good or ill, as a weapon for social change, as a tool for redistributing resources that are inequitably distributed in our society. Only in this way can there be a healthier America over the next fifty years.

It is too much to expect that many of us will be able to break through our self-interest and help lead the struggle for this shift of power and resources. But let us at least try not to stand in the way of such change. And let us not be surprised when those who seek such change—the poor, the elderly, the disabled, endangered workers, prisoners denied health care, the wretched people of the earth and of the United States on whose backs our wealth has been built—defend themselves against us and begin to fight back. As Frederick Douglass, the black abolitionist leader, put it over a century ago: "If there is no struggle, there is no progress. Those who profess to favor freedom and yet deprecate agitation . . . want crops without plowing up the ground. They want rain without thunder and lightning. They want ocean without the awful roar of its mighty waters." There may indeed be a healthier America over the next fifty years, but if *all* our people are to be included, it will require structural changes in our health services and concomitant thunder, lightning, and profound economic and social change.

References

Delgado, M. 1979. "Puerto Rican Folk Healers in the Big Cities." *Forum on Medicine* (American College of Physicians) (December).

Geiger, H. J. 1957. "Social Responsibility of the Physician." *The Scientific Monthly* 85, no. 2 (August).

———. 1976. "The Tasks of Community Medicine." *The Sciences* (New York Academy of Sciences) 13, no. 3 (May/June).

Sidel, V. W. 1979. "Public Health in International Perspective: From 'Helping the Victim' to 'Blaming the Victim' to 'Organizing the Victims.'" *Canadian Journal of Public Health* 70 (July/August).

COMMENTS OF A PRACTICING PHYSICIAN
Malcolm C. Todd, M.D.
Former President, American Medical Association

I have always felt that medicine—the American Medical Association, state medical societies, and all of us in the health industry—will be remembered for what it does in the scientific and social fields in contrast to its endeavors in the political arena. However, we didn't go into the political field of our own free choosing. We were forced into it by politicians and planners, partly to protect our own interests, but also to protect the American public from bad, costly legislation devised for political expediency.

Physicians and the profession must demonstrate more concern for the social and human causes of poor health. Poverty remains the number-one deterrent to good health; unemployment and illiteracy are contributing factors. These are not medical in origin; they are social deterrents to a healthy community. Abuse of alcohol and drugs, obesity, inadequate exercise and other unhealthy behavior not controllable by physicians are also causes of illness and disability.

The time is long past when specific programs of preventive care should have been in operation. Certainly preventive care should involve more than routine immunizations; even in the United States we are deficient as a nation in upgrading immunizations, particularly those for newborn infants and children not yet covered by health insurance. Much of preventive care comes about through the development of sophisticated and realistic programs of health education for all segments of society. It does seem possible that in due time, good prevention should reduce the ultimate cost of health care.

I find myself in agreement with Dr. Geiger on many points. I think that we should look to the future for new prototypes of health care delivery. I have no quarrel with his goals. They are good, and we should try to develop many of them. But, realistically, they can't all be achieved. Making health care accessible to everyone, for example, is an almost impossible goal. I doubt that a compulsory national comprehensive health insurance plan is going to provide access to health for all. Certainly it hasn't, even when mandated, in the socialized nations of the world, including England, Scandinavia, Russia, and even China. For many years, I have advocated putting all citizens in "mainstream medicine." But this has been found to be impractical and unachievable because it simply costs too much. There isn't enough money, even in the United States.

Through community medicine—or perhaps community health is a better term—we should develop and pursue innovative programs to improve the health of all our people. The health team concept is one such program. We must try to provide primary care in areas of poverty and deprivation. As a pilot project this might be done by health workers, or "physicians' extenders," rather than physicians. They would, or could, provide first-line, necessary medical care, working under the supervision of professionals. Their training would have included management of emergency procedures and how to make responsible decisions about entering patients into the health care delivery system.

This is not to advocate the "barefoot doctor" of the People's Republic of China (who, by the way, is neither barefooted nor a doctor), even though that system does work in China. I believe we truthfully can say there is a like need in some areas in the United States, and it should be tried in some of the underprivileged ghettos and slum areas of our inner cities. During the late 1960s attempts were made to develop neighborhood health centers and "free" clinics. Some were effective, but when they failed it was because of administrative inefficiencies or lack of funding, and in some cases, fraud or corruption. If these sound a bit like socialistic programs, they are. But if they work, they would be fulfilling a community health need. Such programs cannot be successful, however, without capital, and more pilot programs should be undertaken. These are not really medical problems. They are social problems, and they could be modified if transportation were made available, along with home care programs, baby sitters, family planning, and education on the harmful effects of repeated pregnancies.

Unfortunately, some planners use infant mortality and life expectancy as indices of the effectiveness of a nation's health care delivery system. But statistics are comparatively meaningless unless the standards and the criteria that are used for measurement are the same for every nation. For example, a birth certificate is issued in the United States if just one breath is taken, whereas in Russia and some Scandinavian countries, and in some other parts of Europe, birth certificates may not be issued unless the infant lives for three, or even six, months. Moreover, how can you equate infant mortality figures in a homogeneous society of 8.5 million in Sweden, with a mixed or heterogeneous, multiple-race society of 225 million, as in the United States? Our infant mortality in Wisconsin and Minnesota, where the Scandinavian population is great, is lower than it is in Sweden.

We can, and we must, do better, and do more to improve the health care of the poor as well as the affluent. It is morally wrong that poor housing, poor nutrition, and poor medical care do exist for some. The fact that it always has existed and always will is no reason we should not try our best to adjust to the need and correct these inequities whenever and wherever possible. I agree that physicians must extend themselves more in community health, and thereby seek to improve the quality of life of all our people.

III EDUCATION AND RESEARCH

6 EDUCATING PHYSICIANS FOR THE FUTURE

Walsh McDermott, M.D.
Senior Adviser, Robert Wood Johnson
Foundation

Walsh McDermott is emeritus professor of Public Health and Medicine, Cornell University, and since 1972, senior officer of the Robert Wood Johnson Foundation. His early research was in microbial diseases and he participated extensively in developing the present-day treatment of syphilis, typhus and typhoid fevers, bacterial pneumonias, and tuberculosis. His later research activities have concerned cross-cultural transfer of technology at home and abroad. These include a complex of studies of health care sponsored and supported by the Navajo Tribe. For the past seven years in his Foundation work, he has been concerned full-time with health care issues in the United States. He is co-editor of the Beeson-McDermott Textbook of Medicine, *a member of the American Academy of Arts and Sciences, a member of the National Academy of Sciences, and a fellow (Hon.) of the Royal College of Physicians (London).*

Most of the time when we need a physician, we don't need a very good one. The need for a high-quality physician usually comes only rarely, or perhaps never. But its coming is wholly unpredictable; it may come tonight for any one of us. And when it comes, if the moment is not properly seized, if a quality physician is not there, or if it not be appreciated in proper time that he or she should be there, the result can be disastrous. The catch is the only person who can really tell you whether you need a middling-to-poor physician or a good physician *is* a good physician. Thus, medical education, as it concerns physicians, must occupy itself entirely with the development of graduates of high quality. This is not to say that we should not have various types of physicians' assistants, but they must be just that. The present discussion, therefore, is concerned with the education of physicians to a high level of quality—to be good physicians.

What do we mean when we say that a person is a good physician? What we mean is that the person can be trusted. As one cannot reasonably be expected never to make a mistake, by "trusted" is meant that there is a high degree of probability that this physician will provide care of high quality in a roughly determinable set of circumstances. In short, an all-important self-discipline is present. The great vital principle—the secret if you will, of medical education and training at its highest quality—lies not in impressive facilities or glittering diagnostic apparatus, but in this deep-seated tradition of self-discipline. For unlike the development of skills in other learned professions, the part of medicine that has to do with the clinical examination of the patient yields an almost exact return for the effort put into it. The key is thoroughness, invariable thoroughness, and as the affair is usually conducted in private, there is no one to monitor the physician's thoroughness. Well aware of this fact, and aware that the probabilities are such that one could get away with time-saving omissions without discovery—at least in the short run—the physician must have been so deeply convinced that he or she bears an inviolable responsibility for thoroughness that any lapse is the equivalent of a conscious, harmful act to someone given into his or her trust.

This is what one cannot see simply by watching another physician's acts—this meticulousness, the sense of always exploring every nook and cranny of the problem. *This acquisition of the deep conviction of the essentiality of thoroughness is the most important feature of the education given in a medical school.*

How is this self-discipline transmitted? By long tradition, the physicians who carry the major responsibility for clinical teaching have this attribute, and they spend much of their time imprinting it in the students. They will constantly reiterate that no excuses are acceptable: The student, once become a physician, has the responsibility for other human beings and when called upon must exercise professional skills just as effectively at three o'clock in the morning as at three o'clock in the afternoon. The major sins, perhaps the greatest, are those termed "sins of omission," wherein the physician cuts a corner and because of fatigue, laziness, or sense of time pressure, fails to perform some examination or obtain some test, and as a result of the omission a patient has been harmed. Medical teachers are quick to spot such professional lapses in a patient's story and (privately of course) hold them up as horrible examples to the student.[a] To imprint medical students (so that it lasts a professional lifetime) with this self-discipline is not something that can be done in casual contacts or a few lectures. It requires that some member of the faculty have steady, repeated contact with the students. Moreover, teaching of this sort does not show up in the complicated calendars of the curriculum. It is a question of reinforcement in the B. F. Skinner (1953) sense, and it requires a considerable amount of time.

It would be idle to pretend that all graduates have this self-discipline or have it to the same degree. But the thought that one's omission might lead to the premature death or permanent invalidism of another person is a powerful persuader, and through the years I have become convinced that virtually all graduates have self-discipline to some degree, and most have it considerably more than that.

While outside observers of this educational activity can see the various aspects of behavior, they are seldom able to perceive this central force of the process. This was well brought out in the decade or so after World War II, when U.S. medical schools—then with high international prestige—were heavily visited by foreign physicians seeking to learn our methods. In my judgment, these visitors, like so many critics of medical ed-

---

[a] In a subtle way, this meticulousness, if overstressed, can have the effect of frightening the young physician away from the general forms of medical care toward the more limited and hence "safer" specialty; likewise it is responsible in part for the overperformance of laboratory tests for "completeness."

ucation today, almost invariably missed the key point of the self-discipline, because it was invisible to them.

I emphasize the point that this quality is invisible, and for this reason one cannot learn to be a physician simply by watching another physician's acts. Of even greater importance is the fact that the self-discipline cannot be measured by written examination or indeed by any *single* examination. There is really no way it can be determined except by observation of the student or physician in action over a considerable period of time. In effect, this is what is done in the last two, all-clinical years of medical school, and also in the several years of residency thereafter. It is on the basis of such observation over two years or so that the faculty or the hospital attending staff can say that someone is a good doctor. As physicians cannot do this when they meet a strange physician, they do the next best thing—they set great store by where that physician received education and training.

There are two other features critical to a high-quality medical education: the clinical clerkship, in which the student serves officially as a very junior physician; and the way basic science is reinforced in the teaching of clinical medicine.

The first clinical clerkships, using medicine, surgery, and pediatrics, represent an entirely different aspect of a medical student's experience and one that is considerably revealing about future abilities as a physician. For it is in these clerkships that the student first attempts to "put it all together." Up until that time the learning process and, indeed, the ability of the medical teachers to devise meaningful examination are essentially the same as in other parts of the university or in the prebaccalaureate college. With the clerkship, however, the constant— that is, daily—confrontation with the living case method puts the student into essentially the same situation that will be experienced throughout the rest of his or her professional lifetime. The student on a hospital service thus bears essentially the same relationship to the patient in bed as does a physician of any age. The student is, of course, clumsy and is much more highly supervised. Thus, with due recognition that all parts of the educational process are interrelated, and hence important, the clinical clerkship in medicine is the most important one.

Much of what is learned in this clerkship is essential to work in surgery, pediatrics, and psychiatry, as well as in medicine. This part of the clinical education has generality for all clinical experience. It is essential for the initial stages of the clerkship that the teaching environment be of the highest quality, because clinical habits get started at that point. Later in the medical student's education—once a high-standard clerkship has been experienced—this is not so important, because by now the student is usually capable of recognizing lapses from high-quality practice.

The student of medicine and the eventual physician have an important knowledge of a number of basic sciences. This is not so that they can do research, which is something erroneously portrayed in the popular press. It is so that they can understand what is wrong with their patients and maintain a constant capability to absorb new methods as they are invented. Medical students must study science, yet they did not really opt for a career in science. Thus, in the initial study of these sciences, the student has to take it on faith that they will become important. The students do the best they can, but it is not an entirely satisfactory process. However, when, toward the end of the second year and at the beginning of the third, they start getting their first individualized clinical experience, they then experience the exciting exercise of seeing how their knowledge of science can be applied to help alleviate, if not totally solve, the problems of their patients. This is a very exciting business and sends them back right away for a better grounding in the particular point in science that was related to a particular patient on a particular day. In short, it's the reinforcement principle of B. F. Skinner. What they are learning by this process is not science per se, for they are not to become scientists. What they are learning is how the clinical physician uses science for the benefit of sick people. If one is to have good general practitioners—or indeed, any sort of physician in today's world—they need to be far more comfortable in the uses of science than was the case even a decade or so ago.

What are the accomplishments and shortfalls of this system? It is highly appropriate that we use the past fifty years as our field of vision because the major forces responsible for the transformation of American medicine and its educational system first became operative at the period's start. Clearly, during these fifty years, U.S. medical schools, considered as a whole, have done a splendid job in turning out graduates and residents who have the built-in capacity to adapt to whatever the future might bring in the way of technologic innovations. This has been shown over and over again. Moreover, through large-scale programs of biomedical research, the medical schools have done a superb job in expanding the knowledge base of medicine and, along with the pharmaceutical and other industries, have developed the interventionist technologies.[b] Thus a good job has been done in generating much new knowledge and transferring that knowledge and the ways to use it to physicians caring for patients during their serious illnesses in hospitals. The medical educational system has not done an equally good job in teaching the ways to use that knowledge for the care of the ambulatory patient. In addition, there is a running debate as to whether there has been a lessening of the emphasis on human support and too much emphasis on the uses of the technologies. There is probably some truth here, but nowhere near what is claimed by medicine's critics. And for well over a decade, efforts to improve the teaching of the Samaritan side have been widespread.

There is certainly another shortfall, not attributable to the medical school per se but certainly attributable to medical educators considered as a single establishment, and that is the divorce between the medical schools and the schools of public health, which occurred just before the fifty-year period of our present focus (Curran 1970). The education of the medical student was thereby impoverished. Because medical students did not learn about public health, the recruitment of that arm of medicine and the professional expertise to focus on people as a group were effectively cut off. As a consequence, despite the generally good job done in turning out graduates capable of handling the unforeseeable technologic future, the schools have done poorly in graduating people able to look at the sys-

---

[b] All the diagnostic, therapeutic, prognostic, and preventive methods, apparatus, and practices whose application affects the course or occurrence of disease with a high degree of predictability.

tem as a whole and hence serve as leaders for further adaptation and change. By a historic coincidence, this separation of medicine and public health happened at the very time research started the marvelous flow of useful products that created the need for the scientifically sophisticated, university-based medical center. The center thus became not something that looked at all of medicine, but something that was a superb instrument for just one of medicine's two parts—the part that has to do with the treatment of individual patients one at a time.

What of the future of this splendid instrument? Along what lines is it likely to develop? To a certain extent, useful answers would require forecasts of what both medicine and our national culture will be like decades hence. Viewed another way, however, one can identify now several major issues with which our medical education will be concerned. Most of these are professional in nature, and some may not assume great prominence for a few decades. There is one issue, medical school financing, however, that if not properly resolved now, could lead in the long run to an important deterioration of the quality of our medical care.

Oddly enough, this is not the usual type of financial situation that will go bankrupt and cease to operate unless more money is forthcoming. The money will be forthcoming. The threat, and it is a major one, is that the ways it is brought in to meet the deficit can get out of hand and seriously damage the intellectual core of the whole enterprise. More specifically, there is real danger that in turning the faculty from teaching and research to the practice of medicine, there is a serious loss of effective teaching time, further exacerbated by the overuse of hitherto inexperienced practitioners as teachers. The other income-generating device—raising the tuition—introduces rigidity into the system. Because of the resulting large indebtedness, payable in dollars or years of indentured service, the young graduates are strongly influenced to choose the most lucrative branches of the profession, in many cases against their instincts and future career desires. In short, the system is facing its most serious threat in fifty years. What makes the threat so serious is the fact that, like moderate exposure to ionizing radiation, the inner deterioration of the medical education might not show for at least as long as a decade. Because the medical schools' adaptations are triggered by economic causes, for the most part they offer economic solutions. Yet an adaptation that just makes the books balance in fiscal terms could be one quite devastating to the educational substance.

We must realize that the economic challenges that have made these adaptations necessary are in large measure not failures of our society but the natural evolution of great social gains. Throughout the years a significant portion of the costs of medical education has come in unidentified form from somewhere else. The attending physicians who were the major clinical teachers of the World War I era received no direct financial support for their extensive work in medical care and teaching on either the inpatient or outpatient hospital services. Appointment to the former was prestigious and intellectually rewarding and was valuable continuing education. Work in the outpatient service was less so, but such an appointment was nevertheless valued because only through it could the professional, and economic, privilege of caring for one's private patients in the hospital be obtained. In addition, such an appointment was a recognized stepping-stone to the prized inhospital attending-physician role. A quite important portion of the education and training effort, and also the medical care itself, thus did not show up as a direct cost. When, in the twenties, the practice of having a few full-time physicians in the clinical faculty was introduced and expanded, they were also the physicians conducting most of the research, and they could get partial support from that source. This practice greatly expanded with the marked increase in the medical school research effort in the two decades following World War II.

Thus a large number of the clinical teachers of medical students, and the supervisors and senior consultants to the residents, did not appear in the educational budget. This fact, coupled with the fact that, generally speaking, the patients involved were nonprivate, gave the clinical department chairmen great flexibility in staffing their teaching programs. With due regard for the patients' welfare, the whole enterprise could be set up along the lines of what was best for teaching. Indeed, the principal factor deciding the better clinical assignments was the physician's reputation as a teacher. It must be noted that throughout that period, say up to 1965, medical leaders believed, and with some cause, that the quality of teaching and that of medical care were inseparable. But the growth of third-party payment—starting with Blue Cross and Blue Shield and expanded with Medicare and Medicaid—changed all that.

Third-party payment, private and governmental, has represented a great social gain in spreading medical care to a very large proportion of our population. This has been accomplished in the face of a population increase from 122.7 million in 1930 to about 223 million today. Understandably enough, a continued expenditure of this size, with a considerable part in public funds, required precise accountability. This has had two strong effects on the educational effort: First, to a considerable, but not yet total, extent, the patients are no longer nonprivate patients; and second, a pernicious doctrine (in the eyes of the educator) has been introduced—namely, the separation of the costs of medical care from those of education.

With these attempts to attain greater precision in the identification of costs has come the need to identify the patient-physician relations; and this linkage of a particular patient to a particular physician has subtly changed the relation of the resident to the patient. The private service and what were formerly the wards or teaching services became the same, in a functional sense. The single factor that previously separated a private from a nonprivate patient was the form of relationship to the physicians. With private patients, the physician who directed their care while in the hospital was someone of their own choice and usually had been their physician before hospitalization, and the residents served as that physician's highly trained deputies. With nonprivate patients it is a physician in the heirarchy of residents who directs the care, and the senior attending physicians and departmental chairmen serve as readily available consultants. Obviously, all these interpersonal relationships have some room for variability, and in the late sixties and very early seventies it was possible to interpret the linkages broadly. As the costs have mounted, the accountability of the linkage has been more strict, to the point that both medical students and residents have to obtain all their clinical experience with what are, in effect, private patients. Without going into the details of what are complex relationships, it is sufficient to say that whereas such a situation can be made reasonably acceptable for the education of the medical students, it considerably dilutes what the residents need most of all at that stage—the opportunity to exercise full *responsibility* without jeopardizing the patient.

The quantitative aspects of the recent and projected fiscal challenges to the medical schools and the adaptations they must make have been well analyzed by Rogers (1979) in his Alan Gregg Lecture for the Association of American Medical Colleges. Selected aspects of the problem have also been presented this year by the Council of Teaching Hospitals (1979) and by Zuidema (1979). From these analyses, and from observations of the pattern employed in the creation of new medical schools, it may be seen that the schools and their allied major hospitals possess only a few mechanisms of response, and they have attempted to activate them all. Except for the use of large increases in tuition, both the public and the private schools have responded in the same ways. The major thrusts on the part of the schools have been a considerable expansion in the use of income from the practice of medicine, a substantial increase in tuition (private schools only), and, for new schools, the substitution of a small group of community hospitals for a major teaching hospital. On the part of the hospital, one response has been to tighten the patients' linkage to the physicians; another has been the divestiture of financial responsibility for anything labeled "teaching," in order to conserve out of the results of the reimbursement rate negotiated the maximal funds to cover operating costs.

Expansion of practice plans and the essentially exclusive use of the off-site clinical campus are responses that are neither good nor bad in themselves. When misused, either one or both can impair the integrity of the education. One might say that the former presents all the problems of the teacher as practitioner, and the latter the problems of the practitioner as teacher.

Considering the last-named first, one way to read the future is to see what has already been happening. Since the beginning of 1968, twenty-nine new medical schools have been opened; twenty-five of them have no major teaching hospital but depend for clinical facilities on affiliation with a consortium, or "ring," of community hospitals. To be sure, several of the group represent second or third medical schools set up within a state in which the initial medical school is united with a major teaching hospital. However, this has little relevance for the medical students in the new schools, most of which are located at some distance, in another city or community. Consequently, all twenty-five of the new schools can be considered together. Since they now make up approximately 20 percent of the nation's medical schools, their emergence as a model must be taken seriously. The actual concept of having a medical school without primary clinical facilities is by no means new. Harvard in a sense followed this formula until the Peter Bent Brigham Hospital was built early in this century, and Northwestern followed the formula for many years. But since the late 1960s, when the Michigan State M.D.-granting school was founded, the trend has been almost all in this direction.

One factor favoring the development was that in many localities in which a medical school was desired there was already a sufficient number of hospital beds, but there was no one hospital to become the major teaching affiliate. Given such a situation, it could be considered irresponsible to saddle the community with the additional beds involved in the creation of a major teaching hospital for the school, to say nothing of the "town and gown" health care struggle that would inevitably be produced. The great significance this strong trend in medical school structure might have for the future lies in the example it presents for all schools of a possible alternative to the close union with a major teaching hospital. Because of obsolescence, a number of these hospitals are facing rebuilding, and for them the issue must be decided fairly soon.

To the school, the principal attraction of the community hospital approach as opposed to the close union with a major teaching hospital is that it takes the school out of the hospital business, so to speak, except for certain clearly specified activities involved in a term-limited contract. From the nature of the situation, the contractual arrangements with any one hospital are small relative to the total operation, so that, conceivably, if a particular affiliation proves unsatisfactory, it can be terminated in good time and another hospital substituted. The concept holds forth the vision of clearly separating health service costs, with the prospect that those costs would turn out to be relatively small and hence manageable. In effect, the vision raises the prospect that one can have a medical school without having to erect a large academic medical center.

A second argument in favor of the community route is that the educational and training experience of the medical students in this setting is more relevant to their own, and society's, future needs than is apt to be the case in a large major teaching hospital.

Examination of these arguments should be prefaced by the statement that there is nothing intrinsic to the teaching of clinical medicine that would prevent its being well done through the community hospital contract formula, provided all concerned are willing to put enough time and money into the effort. By the same token, there are factors in the situation as it is usually constituted at present that can form obstacles to the development of a satisfactory educational program. Some of these factors are subtle, and the probability is great that by no means all have been identified. It is highly appropriate to identify and characterize whatever factors we can, however, with the thought that by relevant modifications in contractual arrangements it might be possible to remove them as obstacles.

Major factors are: the necessity for inserting a cadre of full-time or hospital-based teachers recruited nationally on the staff of the community hospital; the need to develop physicians for the existing staff who would be willing to take on, in addition to their private practice, the quite heavy assignment of training themselves as clinical teachers; the separation of the medical students and residents from the medical school's science base, and frequently from all the research of the clinical departments; the difficulty in obtaining enough patients for the earliest clinical courses—for example, physical diagnosis; and the use of patients closely linked to a wide range of private physicians as a base for the clinical clerkship of medical students and the principal training of residents, including surgical residents.

What it comes down to is that a hospital environment and professional staff that are ideal for the care of all but the most complicated problems do not ipso facto provide a satisfactory base for a clinical clerkship, particularly the initial clerkship. Many of the physicians on the hospital staff may be ideal for "spot teaching," but few, if any, have usually had the training and experience to be professional teachers, nor have they the time or inclination to change their lives to the extent necessary to become professionals. Thus core faculty, usually recruited nationally, must be inserted in the hospital staff in positions of some authority, in most instances as chiefs of service. With today's reliance on medical practice to pay faculty salaries, these newcomers are competitors of the existing hospital staff, in an economic sense as well as on other counts. Both jobs—practice and teaching—require much time. Moreover, the same need for continuity of the physician with patients applies also to physicians' relationships to students. To be sure, an individual member of the practicing profession can make important contributions to the teaching program, but only if there is an organized matrix into which he can fit. He and his fellow practitioners, taken together, are not in a position to create, organize, and maintain that program, even though he can make important inputs to its central philosophy and key contributions to its operation within the very real constraints of his daily responsibilities to his patients. Clinical teaching of medical students, like preclinical teaching, is a highly professional affair—that is to say, in its initial stage it is. Of two equally competent physicians, one may be a splendid teacher, while the other may not be.

These issues must be resolved if the "medical school without walls" concept is to be used to graduate physicians of sufficiently high quality for the future. Legislators definitely acquire the notions that the available practicing profession make an ideal faculty "more in touch with reality" and that the common illnesses of the community hospital offer an educational experience to the medical student superior to the allegedly esoteric disease and illness pattern of the academic medical center. Both notions betray a grave misunderstanding of how an acceptable medical education process works. Yet when a medical school is founded on such notions, with the expectation that an appreciably less expensive education can be maintained, it may take a period measurable in years to establish that its graduates are not satisfactorily educated and trained.

This is a prime danger. Academic leaders in those schools whose clinical teaching is wholly, or almost wholly, conducted off-site must maintain a much closer watch over the teaching program in all its aspects than is done in the schools in which the off-site campus is used to enrich clinical teaching, while the initial clerkships are conducted in primary teaching hospitals. A key point in this close watch is to be sure an adequate investment is being made to convert the community hospital to one appropriate for the initial clerkships. The medical school without walls is a wholly viable concept, but it requires considerably more money than is first imagined, and it must not be sold as a way to provide good medical education "on the cheap."

The point was made earlier that the strict negotiation of reimbursement formulas was to some extent having the effect of making the inpatient services of the teaching hospital and the community hospital resemble each other. Not surprisingly, therefore, certain of the problems of the practice plan—interphysician stresses for example—are similar to those identified for the off-site clinical campus programs. Generally speaking, however, the danger to medical education from practice plans comes from elsewhere. It comes not from their use, but from the temptation to yield to their overuse.

A practice plan is a formal arrangement whereby the members of a clinical department regularly engage in medical practice, with the fees being collected, usually, by the department and allocated by formula toward faculty salaries and other expenses of the school. The type of arrangement varies from one school to another, especially with respect to ceilings on earnings and the extent to which funds are allocated for expenses outside the department in which they were earned. Departments of medicine and surgery, with their various subspecialties, are the big earners; obstetrics and gynecology are usually considerably less so, and pediatrics and psychiatry generally earn the least. The financial return from a plan depends to some extent on the location of the school. The proportion of income from ambulatory care is usually less in a college-town location than in a city. By the same token, the income from ambulatory care is obviously affected if the urban neighborhood of the school is one considered dangerous for personal safety.

Practice plans are not new in concept. Some of the nation's front-rank schools have had them in operation for a number of decades. Nor are the plans limited to the private schools; most state-supported schools have them. Indeed, the State of California recently introduced a uniform practice plan for all its medical schools that supplanted the various individual plans previously in place.

The income generated by practice plans can be substantial— for example, $12 to $14 million annually. In the private schools this income can be the largest single source of operating funds, rivaling in amount the support obtained from the state in the public schools. By the same token, the practice plan income in the state school is not inconsequential. Thus, in a major source of income largely controllable by the medical school itself, the private and public, or state, schools are more and more resembling each other.

In addition to steady and substantial income there are two other advantages to practice plans: They ensure a teaching faculty concurrent, first-hand experience in the practice of medicine; and, particularly if satellite facilities are involved, the plan could serve as the base for an eventual regionalized system of medical care.

But there are disadvantages, too. They arise mainly from dissatisfaction with either the allocations of money or the amount of faculty time devoted to the generation of income. Turbulence is not at all unusual, particularly during the early phases of a plan. With the older plans—that is, those of about twenty years' standing—despite possible early upsets, a tradition of acceptance appears, and the general workings are reasonably smooth. It would be foolish, however, to overlook the fact that there is a source of divisiveness built into the formula, and it may emerge unless vigilance is maintained.

An important disadvantage of excessive reliance on practice plans has to do with the directorships of the individual divisions of large clinical departments such as medicine and surgery. These are key physicians; in effect they possess the prospecting rights for a particular field, such as disease of the liver. By this is meant that they have the responsibility to advance the knowledge of the subject and the capability to use that knowledge effectively in teaching medical students, residents, research fellows, and senior practicing physicians. They are the true curators; virtually full time should be spent in meeting this responsibility. If they were to fall down on the job, the educational and training experience of considerable numbers of people would be diminished. It takes considerable self-discipline to direct a division well and at the same time assume responsibility for private patients. It can be done, but it is not easy. Ideally, the participation of division heads in a practice plan should be limited to serving as true consultative specialists.

At quite another level, problems may arise when there are separate practice plans for each of the various divisions of a large clinical department. The selection of a new departmental chairman becomes subject to individual veto in a way not customary before the divisions were generating income. Indeed, the introduction of a new chairman begins to resemble the entrance of a new senior partner to a large law firm specializing in corporate law. When this is done a substantial amount of faculty time is diverted from educational time—the expansion and transmission of knowledge—and devoted to the practice of medicine. The net time loss is even greater in the nonsurgical branches such as medicine or pediatrics, for the surgeon must operate to retain certain skills; hence the practice time is not all lost. By contrast, the nonsurgical faculty member has ample opportunity for refreshing skills just by participating in the teaching itself.

Obviously the chief danger the practice plan presents to the educational effort is that it is a thief of time. If the plan is used in moderation and the faculty is large, the educational time sacrificed to generate income is not enough to matter. But if the faculty is small and the needed income large, the operation of the plan can badly cripple the performance of the educational function of the school. For, as will be recalled, it requires much time spent with students in order to be of help as they develop that all-important but invisible self-discipline. Overuse of a practice plan becomes not unlike an episode when I was a boy, living in the country. Someone told us that if we spread newspapers over the chunk of ice in our ice box it would not melt so fast. They were right—the only trouble was the milk went sour.

In this look at the issues that will loom large in future medical education, I have dwelt long on the fiscal question. After a fifty-year successful run, the medical schools now find themselves playing with fire in order to survive. I cannot present a list of crisp actions that could be taken to ward off the evils here. My major argument is that the most important part of medical education—acquisition of the inner discipline of the trustworthy physician—can be seriously injured without its being evident. This can go on for several years, or possibly almost a decade, before it becomes clear that what is being presented to the students is mediocre. And we seem headed on a course in which in order to survive financially we risk downgrading the quality of our effort. About all that can be done at the moment is to keep this danger in the forefront of consciousness; to have a clear idea in advance as to what part of the educational effort we must not give up; and to search for the status of these values every time an institutional response such as a practice plan or off-site clinical campus is reviewed—in short, to "know thine enemy" and try to act on the knowledge.

Key issues of future preoccupation, in addition to the fiscal one, are of two sorts: subjects such as care of the elderly, which are just now getting attention but whose importance will predictably increase; and the continued transformation in the nature of the problems facing the pediatricians—many of them transmedical.[c] The fate of issues such as those involved in disease or illness prevention, or the health problems of Third World nations, is unpredictable. This is not to say these issues will not continue to be of importance, but only that it would not be necessary to change medical education to embrace them. There remain four issues, however, that are perceptible now and are fated, in my judgment, for a large future. These are:

---

[c] Problems such as child abuse or learning difficulties that are not solely, or even largely, medical, but medical in part.

1. The schools will have to come to terms with the area known as public health. This will have to be done at least to the point where there will be some organized activity, including the teaching of medical students, in which the uses of science for people considered as groups and the systems for its applications are explored.
2. There will be major attention to ambulatory care in regard to its professional methods, its financial support, and its teaching. These will form much of an activity that could be termed "R and D in medical practice."
3. There will be an expansion of teaching and research in the human values involved in medicine.
4. There will be what in effect is a brand-new area that I shall call "discriminating medicine."

I shall say little about the issue of public health other than to identify it and indicate that it is inconceivable to me that biomedicine for groups will be separated indefinitely from biomedicine for the individual. Although I do not believe emerging physicians should cover all that is presented in today's schools of public health, they should have enough exposure in the uses of science for the benefit of people in groups that they know this world exists, and what it accomplishes. This should be done if for no other reason than that it is a possible career pathway.

The second area has to do with the greatly increased importance of ambulatory care. The dramatic change in the disease pattern during the past five decades has been the substitution of nonmicrobial for microbial disease as the primary condition requiring treatment. The greater proportion of patient visits in an office or other ambulatory care facility is by those who have as their primary condition a chronic disease. (It must be recalled that it is the disease process that is chronic, not necessarily the illness to which it may give rise.)

In the past, there has been almost a complete failure of the educational establishment to work out satisfactory ways of teaching clinical medicine in the care of the ambulatory patient; more recently there have been obvious shortcomings in the system of care itself. There are several reasons for this.

First, in the early part of the century, the knowledge of practical application for the treatment of the patient in hospital and in the office was largely the same. Thus, at completion of the residency, the capability to manage the problems of in-hospital patients could be easily adapted to the problems of patients seen in the office. But the technology has increased by leaps and bounds. Some of it—at first, at least—could be managed only in the hospital. And the ways in which it could be adapted for use on an ambulatory basis were not systematically pursued. Indeed, diseases thought at the beginning of the period to mandate hospitalization imperatively, such as tuberculosis and pneumonia, were altered by the technology so that they could be managed at home, or even to some extent on an ambulatory basis.

In a real sense, ambulatory care has failed to keep up with the technologic revolution and hence has developed no new systems through which the technology can be applied. Examples are such issues as how to ensure that asymptomatic patients leading normal lives should self-administer medications daily over periods of weeks or months; how to have some sort of answering service whereby they can learn out-of-hours if they are proceeding correctly; and how to teach them to perform various sets of exercises faithfully and know when it is advisable to skip them. Matters such as these, and some considerably more complex, cannot be influenced over a period of months by the physician's piercing glance and unforgettable words in a twenty-minute office interview.

Our slowness to recognize how the technology has changed the conditions under which ambulatory care must operate is one side of the problem. The other is the poor record of the medical school in the teaching of ambulatory care. I have been convinced for some years (McDermott 1971) that the chief cause is the factor of *time* in relation to the evolution of disease and illness in ambulatory patients. A medical student caring for a patient in a hospital bed is in the same situation that he will be in throughout his professional life when caring for a hospitalized patient. The biologic events in that patient show rapid change—sometimes in a minute, sometimes in days, or a week or so. Moreover, because it is within the hospital, the student can witness these changing events himself, if need be in the evenings and on Sundays. Thus it is relatively easy to fit an intense and exciting educational experience into the time constraints of the schedules of an educational program. The inpatient clinical clerkship is thus a first-class teaching simulator. Indeed it is better than a simulator; it is the situation as it exists in the real world.

By contrast, change for better or worse in ambulatory patients may not occur for months, or an interval long beyond the period that would fit any reasonable curriculum. It is also difficult to extend the teaching sessions in ambulatory care to include nights, as is so easily done with the inpatient clerkship. Yet really to get the true experience, it would be necessary to work, or at least be on call, for longer periods than the conventional outpatient clinic is open. To stimulate real-world conditions, it would be necessary for students or doctors to immerse themselves completely in ambulatory care for a considerable period—for example, nine months to a year. As a practical matter, therefore, it is not really possible within the time constraints of a reasonable predoctorate medical education to give students true experience in ambulatory care. And the hit-and-run type is enough to imprint them with the desire to stay as far away from it as possible.

Corrections of this shortfall will require considerable thoughtful effort, and important beginnings have already been made. Today when the motivation to try to correct this teaching deficiency is high, the medical school is in great danger of losing the facilities in which to do it because of the large financial losses they appear to be producing for the hospital. The sums involved are considerable; two of the best-known such university hospitals in a large city each report annual losses of more than $6 million.

Various ways of rearranging the ambulatory care service are undergoing trial, but with present reimbursement policies, ambulatory care holds little prospect of being anything but a serious loss to the large, private, major teaching hospital. When the medical school tries to ameliorate its financial problems by creating a practice plan, the problem is exacerbated because those ambulatory patients whose care *is* reimbursable are drawn into the medical school plan, leaving for the hospital only the medically indigent group.

We have here another instance in which the adaptation to a financial challenge can serve to damage seriously the quality of the teaching effort. For unless this fiscal drain can be neutralized—presumably by a change in reimbursement policies— it is difficult to see how the major urban teaching hospitals on which private medical school teaching is based can do other than attempt to abandon all ambulatory care services except for those provided through the emergency room. This is the traditional pattern for most community hospitals, the bulk of whose ambulatory medicine is conducted in the private offices of the staffs. As the teaching of clinical medicine with ambulatory patients tends to increase the length of visits, it adds to costs, and hence, unless specially reimbursed, is not a financially attractive proposition to prepaid medical care plans. Thus one of the high-priority assignments of the medical school in the immediate future is not only to improve greatly its ability to teach ambulatory care but above all to find some way in which the care can be funded in a facility that would permit proper student and resident education and training. Parenthetically, it can be stated that in the foreboding university hospital curtailment of ambulatory care, we have a classic example of falling dominos. The academic medical center of which the medical school is a part will be called upon to play a critical extramural role in the future. Yet by far the principal instrument a hospital has for any kind of outreach program is the capability to provide ambulatory care.

The third area for future consideration has to do with values in human support that I have come to label, "Samaritanism." There are many aspects to this subject, but there are two points of importance to the medical education of the future: First, we are gradually recognizing that a very large portion of today's Samaritanism is actually technologically based. Second, we are just beginning to realize that the notion that one can teach these matters by example is a fallacy. I have tried to describe this function elsewhere (McDermott 1978:)

> ... the Samaritan function has a number of aspects. In the last analysis it can be defined as the diagnosis and treatment of the patient's illness, as opposed to his disease. By, "the illness," is

meant what the patient is experiencing and by "the disease," what he has. Based on compassion, Samaritanism is by no means simply an exercise in love; its proper performance also requires a mastery of science and technology. In large measure but not yet in toto, Samaritanism is an indirect but nevertheless real use of science and technology. For over the long pull, the greatest effect of Samaritanism lies in reassurance—in human support. Sometimes the reassurance can be quickly and decisively delivered; sometimes it takes more time.

I think most of us would agree that a patient's primary feeling when he seeks medical care is an intense wish to find out that whatever it is that is wrong, it is not something that will cause him awful harm. Lower on the priority list is curiosity as to the precise nature of what may be wrong, it is not something that will cause him awful harm. This is really a matter of secondary interest. But for one human being to make the judgment about another that whatever is wrong is not a serious threat and make that judgment stick requires that the judge, in this case the physician, have a legitimatizing base. Prior to fifty years ago, the legitimatizing base for such judgments and the reassurance they formed, was really mostly dogma—a dogma mellowed and well polished by experience. Today's doctor derives his legitimatizing base, the base that permits him to dispense reassurance, from his expertise in the use of a broad spectrum of scientific and technical knowledge.

I do not believe this point of the major role our technology plays in strengthening the human factor, or Samaritan function, of medicine has been well recognized. It has real implications for the educational process of the future. One may say kindness cannot be taught. Perhaps so—but kind ways of communicating the results of our science-based tests can be taught. Sometimes that base for reassurance is obtained promptly. But how about the cruelly long interval between biopsy and the pathologists's report? Again, the result may provide wonderful reassurance, but the patient may have gone through quite an ordeal in the interval.

The other point about the Samaritan function in education has been that for some years now we have deluded ourselves that we teach it by example, long after the spread of modern hospital architecture has served to prevent us from doing so. We were teaching this side of medicine by example when I was a young teacher, but we seldom do so now. The reason is not hard to find. In the old days the teaching physician operated before the eyes of many in the goldfish bowl of the open ward and was always conscious of the need to represent a fine example of the compassionate physician. Indeed, for most of the patients in the miserable conditions of our city hospitals it was about all the physician had to offer, and he was careful to see that students were imbued with this spirit.

With the far greater privacy afforded the patient today, the situation is quite different. When the teacher is before the students—as contrasted to his clinical care role—he treats the patient courteously, but with a detached courtesy, and he concentrates his teaching on the disease rather than on the illness. But when those moments come when a clinician has to break some awful news or knows that for some other reasons he must go all out in human support, he does not take five or ten medical students with him—*he goes alone* and usually sees the patient in a private room or floor office. Since the students never see this, and since we have been reticent in talking about it, the students have not realized that it occurs. Thus, while we still represent "the example," we have long excluded the students from witnessing our behavior as an example of the compassionate physician.

Once this problem is surfaced, it can be approached in various ways, starting with a lecture or seminar course on the subject for the first-year class. By hiding the human support side from the teaching side, we have been running the risk of producing some physicians who customarily treat the disease but not always the illness it produces, or all of that illness. First-year students, perhaps because they still represent the public more than the profession, can instantly grasp this distinction between the treatment of illness and the treatment of disease. What is more, they claim to be considerably more interested in the treatment of the illness, as they are sometimes convinced the faculty are not. In part, this borders on anti-intellectualism; hence, in the teaching it is necessary to stress the social and human support vaule of the control of the disease as well as the management of illness. But on balance this development is most hopeful. It looks as if merely by surfacing these problems for systematic study early in medical school, we can do a great deal. We can ensure that the student sees the technologic function and the human support function of medicine in proper relation to each other right from the beginning. And what better way is there to educate the doctor of the future?

The fourth of the issues I have chosen as being of great importance in the education process of the future has to do with what some of us are beginning to call the teaching of "discriminating medicine" (Rogers 1979). By this is meant a form of medical practice in which on the diagnostic side all observations and tests are not made at once, but the story is allowed to unfold; the therapy and management side is fitted as carefully as possible to the realities of the individual situation. There is no accepted body of knowledge and practice on this subject available today. Much will have to be done to develop it, and it is here that the research and development in medical practice—a large activity in the future, it is hoped—will have its greatest productivity.

I am convinced that over the long term the technologic imperative will not go away. In fact, I would not wish to see it do so. Human imagination must have full play. But if the technologic imperative will not go away, there certainly will come a time when society cannot tolerate the costs in money, and in the rest of our resources, of virtually unlimited technologic developments in biomedicine. A free society cannot suppress such technologic development, however, and so-called technologic assessment in the strict sense is not very likely to succeed: There is really nothing to assess until the genie is out of the bottle; the process must be interrupted at some other stage. Medical costs—that is, the portion attributable to use of the technology—begin at the bedside or in the physician's office. Therefore, to control these costs, an important influence must be exerted at the time of the first patient-physician encounter, and obviously the only party equipped to do this is the physician.

This physician must be one with a considerable familiarity not only with the many clinical manifestations of the disease but also with the whole panoply of products of the technology that conceivably could be relevant to the situation. From this information, possessed and developed by the physician, *discriminating choices* must be made. Making the choices is imperative, for it is becoming impossible to apply the whole panoply at once or within a short period.[d] To be able to make these discriminating decisions, physicians must operate from a position of inner security, the security provided by possession of the discipline of thoroughness, and by the knowledge that they know enough—that is, have been sufficiently well educated in medicine—to make the proper choice.

In short, we must have better-educated and more finely trained physicians in the future than we have today, which goes squarely against much of the present-day conventional wisdom on how to ensure the widest distribution of satisfactory general medical care. In our effort to do this, many task analyses have been made, along with judgments as to the professional or paraprofessional best fitted for the task. A subtle danger has come to pervade all this activity—namely, the tacit assumption that an acceptable goal would be a physician trained in some practical way that would not require as much attention to the full range of diseases, their illnesses, and the science base as is presently the case. Certainly, continuous review of task assignment among the various groups is an important activity and should be continued. But my reading of the forces emerging for the future is that there will be no way out of this dilemma of the technologic imperative, on the one hand, and the defense of the patient and the taxpayer on the other, *other than through the education and training of physicians of high quality*. The question then arises, is this an academic dream or can it be done?

My answer is that it has been done, specifically in the case of microbial diseases. Broadly speaking, this was the first field to feel the impact of the modern biomedical technology. For a short period following the introduction of sulfonamides, physicians could lead an easy life, in the sense that once they gave sulfonamide to a patient, they could relax in confidence that they had done all that modern science and technology could do for the patient. But life became more complicated: Other antimicrobial drugs were discovered, and it was no longer possible to give them all. And perhaps more important, narrowly spe-

---

[d] Essentially the same force—the rich productivity in technologic development—will lead to some workable solution of the malpractice and defensive-medicine problem.

cific drugs were developed, and they had to be given when the patient was first seen if they were to have full effectiveness. Yet the diagnostic methods of the day would not permit specificity for many hours, perhaps only for as long as a week, following the initial encounter. Given this situation, considerable discrimination obviously had to be employed. The extent to which the discriminatory ability was acquired in the early days undoubtedly varied considerably. Without question, however, this ability exercised on the first encounter was the hallmark of the superior consultant on microbial diseases. Those consultants really had no technologies not readily available to everybody else. What they had was a great knowledge of disease manifestations and relative therapies, organized in the brain in such a way as to provide the capability to make the discriminating choices. Thus it can be done. Basically what these clinical experts in microbial diseases had was that they were better *clinicians*.

It should also be noted that not only does this trend in the direction of a high-quality physician for the future run to some extent against contemporary trends in medical training, but it also creates its own problems in costs. Not infrequently the discriminating process involves performing only a few tests and allowing the situation to unfold before more are done. Thus the actual period in the hospital is lengthened and there must be a trade-off between the costs of more hospital days and those of greater use of the diagnostic and therapeutic technology.

Granting the truth of my prediction that for the future, rather than having less highly trained physicians, they must be more highly trained, how do we teach this discriminating medicine? The acuteness of the dilemma cannot be overemphasized. When the senior physician comes in on a Monday morning to discover that the resident has not ordered a chest film on a particular patient, does he pin a star on the resident for showing fine, educated, discriminatory medicine, or does he upbraid the resident for cutting corners? This is the dilemma— how to teach the student the ability to make discriminating choices without teaching the corner-cutting habits of the undisciplined physician. Although the need can be perceived now, how to do it is far from clear. Nevertheless, there have been some perceptions and there is some research, which I classify as part of the "R & D of medical practice," developing the knowledge we must have for this educational process.

One of these observations is that today's physician to a surprising extent has lost the prognostic ability for the nonsurgical diseases of adults. This is a major "loss"; the term is in quotes because we never actually had it for the diseases encountered now, but we did have it for the diseases that formed the bulk of the physician's practice several decades ago. Proper use of the diagnostic, therapeutic, and preventive tools of medicine—that is, use with discrimination—depends in large measure on the degree of accuracy by which the dangers to the patient in the particular set of circumstances are perceived. Moreover, on the Samaritan side, the ability to forecast is one of the most important things a doctor can do, for it allows the patient, the physician, and any others involved a chance to adjust to, or cease to worry about, what lies ahead. In the choice of therapeutic interventions, the predictable course in the absence of the intervention is obviously of decisive importance. Writing on this problem elsewhere (McDermott 1977: 148), I have said:

So long as the pattern of illness faced by the practitioner in the United States was almost always that of an obvious microbial disease among the younger members of the population, the knowledge on which the ability to forecast was based was reasonably adequate. With most microbial diseases, individual cases all tend to be alike, and the period from onset to full clinical illness is only a matter of days or hours. Under these circumstances, the data supplied in the disease descriptions in textbooks is quite satisfactory. But the U.S. pattern of illness faced by the practitioner today is no longer mainly a matter of obvious microbial disease among the young but of highly diverse hidden structural diseases, frequently with several decades between actual (undetected) onset and outcome. Textbooks of medicine, which can easily communicate the prognosis of measles or rabies with accuracy can provide only the most general sort of information about such maladies as coronary heart disease, rheumatoid arthritis, or cancer of the prostate that today claim the physician's attention. Although a particular chronic disease may be common, its individual expressions may be so diverse as to afford a single physician encounters with

only one or two examples of each expression in his professional
lifetime.

Even though textbooks of medicine cannot encompass all the
recorded medical experience needed for a base of prognosis in
the many variations of coronary heart disease, electronic data
processing can be employed to provide such a data base. And
extensive studies of the use of this method in cardiovascular
disease have been going on for a number of years now by Stead
(1972), and subsequently by Wallace and his associates at
Duke (Rosati et al. 1975). In addition, similarly based studies
on the prognosis of coma have been carried on by Plum et al.
at Cornell. The enormity of the tasks involved in using this
approach for our entire spectrum of diseases can hardly be ex-
aggerated. Nevertheless, the manifestations of at least certain
of the principal diseases can be organized in this way, and
when this is done it will make an important contribution to
our teaching of discriminating medicine for the future. The data base could provide discriminating physicians with instant
access to the almost infinite variety of the subsets of disease of
a single cause. The other type of study I could cite is being
conducted at Yale and has to do with the actual sharpening of
the measurement of the clinical manifestations of disease. This
is the so-called clinicometrics of Feinstein. Its object—and he
can show some useful results—is to sharpen the definition of
various clinical findings so that they can form a data base for
various uses, including prognosis.

I believe I am safe in saying that throughout the past fifty
years there has been relatively little effort in our medical
schools to improve the quality of clinical medicine in the sense
of improving the physician's perceptive ability in the transaction of the first encounter. To be sure, there has been a good
deal of work on history taking. There has really been, however, no effort to meet this important problem of the fallaway in
the base of our ability to forecast the outcome of our patients'
diseases and illnesses. There was one interesting point on the
purely clinical side, presented by Dr. Lawrence Altman in a
signed article in the *New York Times,* about a Dublin physician who had been able to demonstrate that the familiar phenomenon of wrinkled hands following submersion in dishwater

does *not* occur after relevant nerves have been badly damaged. Its appearance, or rather its reappearance, can thus be useful as a measurement of the rate of healing of severed approximated nerves.

As this approach toward the goal of discriminating medicine continues—and I am sure it will—our profession may be able to make the long overdue peace with science with which it and other learned professions collided in the nineteenth century.

As we review the happenings of these past fifty years and attempt to judge what they bode for the future, certain things will stand out which I have sought to identify:

- The fact that an educational effort over considerable time and involving considerable numbers of highly experienced teaching faculty is necessary to transmit the inner discipline that makes the wholly trustworthy, and hence responsible, physician.
- The fact that hospital architecture has removed one of the stages on which we can serve as role models has eliminated a once major opportunity to teach the human support side of medicine by example. We must do it in some other and more systematic way.
- The need to restore at least a small portion of the loss we suffered as a result of the separation of medical education from the schools of public health.
- The great importance of ambulatory care and our present inability to come truly to grips with it, either educationally or fiscally.
- The fact that research and development in medical practice are badly needed in forming a base for prognosis of the illnesses of our adult patients with today's diseases. Indeed, the conscious knowledge that we have largely "lost" this prognostic ability is overdue.
- The warning that in our frantic attempts to finance everything that we now have, in the face of the inflationary challenge, we run a considerable, identifiable set of risks to the substance of our medical education. I suspect that we are at present going through the same gradually crumbling attitudes here as with our other reactions to inflation. At first

we are trying to save everything; ultimately we will recognize that certain things are really not all that important.

So that I may end on a note of the optimism that I feel, let me point out that fifty years ago was the fall of 1929—the beginning of the Great Depression of the 1930s. I started medical school then. I do not propose to discuss the Depression, although like all who survived it as adults, it left a deep imprint on my thinking. Indeed, Caroline Bird named her book on the Depression *The Invisible Scar,* and I have such a scar. But in that book she makes the point that "manufacturing as a whole did not grow at all between 1930 and 1940. Big business remained virtually unchanged . . . All but four of the top ten manufacturing corporations of 1930 . . . ended the decade with fewer assets than they had started with."

I would like to point out that the period when there was no economic growth was the very one in which the two greatest developments in biomedicine of the twentieth century were made, namely, the antimicrobial drugs in the form of prontosil (1935), and the discovery, made then but reported in 1942, that nucleic acid, specifically DNA, was the stuff by which heredity is transmitted.

We will continue to need medical education. The forces developing in the field are such as to demand that education must be of high quality. From a viewpoint supported by the impoverished start of these fifty years, it is clear that the fact that our medical education institutions have to scramble to survive financially does not mean they need be trade schools or anti-intellectual. This will happen only if we let it, by trying to save everything we had at the peak of our golden times. For, and this is the message that those early days in the 1930s have deeply imprinted in me, we must recall that there was another time when we were poor and we had our Camelot, too.

References

Association of American Medical Colleges Council of Teaching Hospitals. 1979. "Toward a More Contemporary Public Understanding of the Teaching Hospital." Washington, D.C.: Department of Teaching Hospitals, Association of American Medical Colleges.

Bates, D. et al. 1977. "A Prospective Study of Nontraumatic Coma: Methods and Results in 310 Patients," reprinted from *Annals of Neurology* 2:3, September.

Curran, J. A. 1970. *Founders of the Harvard School of Public Health, with Biographical Notes 1909-1946.* New York: Josiah Macy, Jr., Foundation.

McDermott, W. 1971. "Do Medical Schools Have to Be Restructured to Produce the Doctor of the Future?" Proceedings of the *Anglo-American Conference on Medical Care,* Royal *Society of Medicine,* London, England, April 5-7.

———. 1978. "Medicine: The Public Good and One's Own" (The Paley Lecture). *Perspectives in Biology and Medicine* 21, no. 2 (Winter).

———. 1977. "Evaluating the Physician and His Technology." *Daedalus* 106, no. 1 (Winter).

Rogers, D. E. 1979. "On Preparing Academic Health Centers for the Very Different 1980s," The Alan Gregg Memorial Lecture, November 5.

Rosati, R. A.; J. F. McNeer; C. F. Starmer; B. S. Mettler; J. J. Morris; and A. G. Wallace. 1975. "A New Information System for Medical Practice." *Archives of Internal Medicine* 135, no. 8 (August).

Skinner, B. F. 1953. *Science and Human Behavior.* New York: MacMillan.

Stead, E. 1972. Presidential address: Transactions of the Association of American Physicians. 85.

Zuidema, G. 1979. "The Impact of Social Change on Medical Education." *The Pharos* 42:4, Fall.

MORE CHANGE AND CHALLENGE FOR MEDICAL EDUCATION
John A. D. Cooper, M.D.
President, Association of American Medical Colleges

A better understanding of the normal processes of living systems and the nature of changes that occur in disease has transferred medicine from an empiric base to a sounder scientific base. Society recognizes that this revolution of the past three decades has greatly increased the capabilities of medicine to make a difference in the quality and length of life. Physicians are expected to employ the full range of these advances in their medical care.

Most patients equate new technology with improvement in health care and expect that it will be employed in the resolution of their medical problems. This attitude makes it difficult to exert controls over the introduction and use of new technology, as the record of the health-planning effort demonstrates. Modern technology, properly used, is an essential component of the thoroughness of Dr. McDermott's good physician.

Perhaps we have led our people to expect too much from medical care. It can make a relatively small contribution to the improvement of the nation's health status. Nutrition, the effects of our environment, and lifestyle are important factors in the well-being of our people, even in the infectious diseases that have occupied Walsh McDermott's attention over several decades. Medical care can make a contribution to health status, but most interventions that really make a difference in the outcome of disease are those that come from the advances flowing from biomedical research. Unfortunately, many of these interventions are complex and expensive.

However, as McDermott points out, patients expect more from their physician than competence in applying modern biomedical knowledge and technology in dealing with their illness. They also expect their doctor to care and be empathetic. This aspect of the art of medicine is not dealt with as effectively as it should be in medical education or by many physicians in their practice. A recent study for the Robert Wood Johnson Foundation found that although only 12 percent of the population surveyed had overall dissatisfaction with their medical care, 28 percent were unhappy with the waiting time to see a physician, 18 percent with the information provided by the physician on what was wrong, 16 percent with the amount of time they spent with the doctor, and 13 percent with the amount of concern the doctor appeared to have about them. Although the feelings expressed by patients do not suggest a large problem with caring and empathy, they do suggest that we need to pay greater attention to the human aspects of medicine. As life becomes more complex and demanding, with the need to adjust to fewer resources and a consequent lowering of our standard of living, patients will need more reassurance and caring from their physicians. Medicine appears to be the only generally available source of support for their anxieties and uncertainties.

The concerns that McDermott raises about the balancing of faculty participation in teaching, research, and patient care are well taken. With the inadequacy of other sources of support to meet rising costs of medical education, the faculty have substantially increased their financial contributions to their institutions by greater involvement in patient care. Medical practice plan income is the fastest growing source of support, and there is little evidence that it will be replaced by other sources in the future unless tuition levels are greatly increased to cover a larger fraction of the costs of medical education. The involvement in more patient care has compromised faculty involvement in teaching and research. In fact, federal research support has fallen from a high of 36 percent of the total revenue of medical schools in 1963–64 to 18 percent in 1977–78. These expenditures serve as a proxy for the change in effort.

With the new balance in faculty effort has come a decrease in the interest of young physicians in a career in academic medicine. If they view a major faculty responsibility to be medical practice, they find little difference in that role and the private practice of medicine, and the financial rewards can be much greater in the latter. Studies by the Association of American Medical Colleges indicate that the declining interest in a faculty career will result in a shortage of full-time clinical faculty in the future. Unless trends are reversed, medical education may again become heavily dependent on volunteer faculty who donate time from their private practice to teaching students. This will have implications for the type of medical education we provide and the role of the medical school in advancing knowledge.

There are other trends in medical education that I believe will become more evident in the future. The changing nature of the sciences basic to medicine and the growth of graduate medical education call for a more effective articulation of the present compartmentalization in premedical, undergraduate medical, and residency education and training programs. Experiments are under way in several universities, with support from the Commonwealth Fund, to integrate university science departments and basic science departments in the medical school.

The graduate phase of medical education has become as important as the undergraduate period. More than 90 percent of our graduates expect to continue in residencies until they have qualified for certification by a specialty board. Graduate medical education has coalesced around the medical schools. Over 95 percent of all residents are in programs sponsored by teaching hospitals associated with medical schools. These developments should be considered an opportunity and a challenge to medical educators. The planned inclusion of educational material and experience better provided during the graduate phase is now possible if faculties begin an interdisciplinary examination of their residency programs.

Continuing medical education is also coming under greater scrutiny. There is evidence that the traditional courses for practicing physicians do not have an important impact on the quality of care they provide. New approaches are centered more on the assessment of a physician's individual needs, with feedback from the monitoring of his practice. All these efforts are directed at rationalizing the continuum of medical education.

Medical education has changed over the past fifty years to keep pace with new knowledge and changing societal needs. They have been halcyon days for medicine, but even greater challenges face us in the future. History has, however, provided ample evidence that the university and its medical school are enduring institutions. They have survived the Inquisition, waves of anti-intellectualism, and despots who would impose their will. They will survive to have their accomplishments reviewed again in the year 2030.

NEW DIRECTIONS IN EDUCATION
Nathan J. Stark
Undersecretary, U.S. Department of Health
and Human Services

We must recognize the need for training physicians to strive for excellence, exemplified by the practice of an inner discipline, for the thoroughness of diagnostic investigation at the crucial time is vital. I also agree with Dr. McDermott that one area where we have not measured up is ambulatory care, and that this is an aspect of medical care that increasingly demands substantial development and refinement. I acknowledge that we have witnessed a widening gulf between medical practice and public health, that medical education should emphasize primary care, preventive medicine, and an expansion of research and training in geriatrics, and that there is substantial value in the trend to organizing the newer medical schools as community-oriented institutions. I believe, perhaps more strongly than Dr. McDermott expresses, that a quality medical education can be fostered without relying on a large teaching hospital connected to the medical school, but I hasten to add that I also concede that the cost of doing this is usually much more than is admitted. The need to inculcate human values into the processes of medical practice is crucial, especially in view of lenghtened lifespans and the nature of care we should be providing to older and chronically ill persons. And I agree that physicians need to be taught to use technology in a more discriminating fashion.

I also believe that the federal government can play an important role in meeting some of the needs that I've just cited, by funding research, disease prevention, geriatrics, and technology assessment, and by providing money for training in primary care, prevention, geriatrics, and cost-effective clinical practice. Recent Department of Health and Human Services activities of note in this regard include the National Center for Health Care Technology and increased support for departments of family medicine and for residencies in primary care in family medicine.

J would place a different emphasis on some aspects of medical care and education, and would disagree with some of Dr. McDermott's conclusions. For example, he seems to dismiss the role of nonphysician health care providers. The discussion of this issue is in one sentence: "That is not to say that we should not have various types of physicians' assistants, but they must be just that." I believe that the extension of care to the millions of people who are inadequately served can be greatly facilitated by a judicious wider use of nurse practitioners and physicians' assistants.

Another example of a different emphasis is a greater recognition that many of the encounters between the patient and the physician are of a routine nature. This does not lead one to want a lower quality of medical preparation, but it does suggest the need to develop more fully a variety of roles, a move that may incidentally reduce cost.

Finally, though Dr. McDermott notes that "expansion of practice plans and the use of the off-site clinical campus are neither good nor bad in themselves," he tends to underscore only the bad aspects, and I would propose a more balanced view.

Of greater concern than these shades of emphasis, however, are two important problems encountered in the preparation of physicians, areas deserving of greater attention. First, one of the vital and growing roles of physicians is as teachers of their patients, especially if we are to succeed in increasing our emphasis on prevention. This role takes on greater significance the more we recognize the importance of personal behavior—lifestyle—to disease avoidance.

Second, at HHS we are shaping programs and budgets to correct a serious imbalance in medical care, improving coverage of those who are medically underserved. There are about 50 million people in rural areas in America and in the inner cities who do not have ready access to a physician for regular medical attention. This problem is relevant to medical education, because we rely on new graduates to fill in these gaps in services by their choice of practice locations. We are finding some ways to make a difference, through the Area Health Education Centers, through the National Health Service Corps and its scholarship program, and through community health care development.

On the whole, I am in accord with the views set forth by Dr. McDermott, and my differences in emphasis are not overriding. I find as perplexing as he does, and as about as insoluble, the general problem of financing medical education. But we are on common ground in seeking well-trained physicians, high-quality ambulatory care, and a greater emphasis on prevention in public health for the entire population.

THE VIEW FROM THE ACADEMIC MEDICAL CENTER
William G. Anlyan, M.D.
Vice President for Health Affairs, Duke University

Every academic administrator in this country ought to look at the 1980s with problems of general economy, inflation, and energy in the forefront. Some of the high-priority programs for health care in the eighties should be genetic counseling, perinatal care, immunization of infants and children, and selected areas for preventive care in adults. We need educational programs to eliminate social habits that tend to cause advanced diseases in later life. We are planning to look at the problems of optimizing outpatient care versus costly inpatient care. We can now put information on coronary patients on computers, sifting out those who can go home in four days from those who need to stay for three weeks at $350–$500 a day. These are some of the innovations taking place in the academic health centers that have repercussions on the cost of health care in the 1980s.

As to the educational process, Dr. Cooper referred to the experiments of the Commonwealth Fund, which provide much greater interface activity between the academic medical center and the collegiate system. These experiments are going on in eight universities. We are still coping with the admission process. We still have too many valedictorians from mediocre high schools who cannot get into the mainstream of medical education, and currently only one out of three applicants for admission to medical school is successful. In particular, we are interested in the qualifications that will augment humanism in medical care.

Regarding capitation support, if we don't have some form of basic, stable financing for the academic medical centers, we will end up as has happened in Japan, where they have public schools for everybody who can gain admission, except the very wealthy. The latter enter the private system of academic medical centers, where the tuition can be as high as $40,000 a year. Now what would be the impact of high tuition on health care in the eighties and nineties? A lot of the young Japanese medical students look upon that $40,000 a year as a pass-through investment that they're going to recoup later on in their practice. We certainly don't want to see that happen in the United States in the future.

We also have skeletons in our closets that need to be cleaned up: For instance, various specialty boards, in isolation, write the type of experiences that their residents need to have. Hand surgery is an example. Is it in the domain of the orthopedic, plastic, or general surgeon? The public is confused as to who does what. We need to define who is qualified to do hand surgery, and the same problem exists in other specialties.

Continuing education is probably going to be the biggest sleeper we've got to address in order to improve health care. Unfortunately, we know only what doesn't work and what is expensive and works well; but we've got to figure out what works optimally in a variety of settings. The solution should include other health professionals, who might form health teams in coronary care units, around renal dialysis, or in intensive-care nurseries. In biomedical research, we certainly hope that it will be more stable—perhaps on a five-year, roll-forward plan, rather than on a "disease-of-the-year" basis.

What should be the role of the federal government vis-à-vis the private sector? I personally feel very strongly that the federal government should intrude only when the private sector is incapable of handling the problems before us. The federal government lacks the long-range planning capability, and too often it falls prey to doing what is politically expedient. It has no institutional memory. For instance, when the amendments for end-stage renal disease were added to Medicare in 1972, did anybody raise a question as to what it would cost or whether it was the nation's number-one priority? Should they have considered putting more money into genetic counseling, perinatal care, and the things that prevent disease at the front end of life, rather than at the end stage of life?

It should be added that we in the private sector are not ourselves pure; to date I would have to admit that we have had some disorganized, fragmented, and adversarial factions. But the private sector is now beginning to work together and to look at these issues on a long-range basis. Our future depends on the stable support of biomedical research, and it is my fond hope that this might be pegged to some percentage of national health expenditures, as is done in most major industries, so that once and for all we will get past the point of bargaining and pleading for a budget year by year.

7 THE OUTLOOK FOR BIOMEDICAL RESEARCH

James A. Shannon, M.D., Ph.D.
Former Director, National Institutes of Health

Dr. James A. Shannon was director of the National Institutes of Health when funding for medical research increased year after year, reaching $2 billion a year, with the NIH portion of these expenditures accounting for 40 percent of the whole. Under his administration, research and training grants for universities provided a clear demonstration that there could be a blending of the public interest with academic research without interference to scientific progress. His influence in the promotion of medical research not only brought improvement to the medical centers but led to many improvements in health care for the populace. A contributing editor and writer of articles for professional journals, Dr. Shannon, born in Hollis, New York in 1904, has been in the forefront of research activity almost from the start of his career in 1931 as an assistant in the Department of Physiology at the New York University College of Medicine. His activities have included directorships in the research service of the New York University medical division, the Squibb Institute of Medical Research, and the National Institutes of Health. A founding member of the advisory committee on medical research for the Pan American Health Organization, Dr. Shannon also has served as a consultant to the U.S. Surgeon General and to the President's Science Advisory Committee, and as vice chairman of the standing committee of the Federal Council on Science and Technology.

There will be many changes in the nation's biomedical research programs in the years to come, though perhaps not as extensive as those that have taken place in the last half-century. But one thing is certain now, and that is that to have continuing excellence and high productivity, the changes must provide for

1. Strengthening of the infrastructure of the biomedical sciences
2. Stabilization of the institutions where the research and the research training effort are located
3. A more visible set of career opportunities than obtain today
4. Continuous renewal of both manpower and physical resources

These conditions of operation are imperative if the biomedical sciences are to serve their ultimate purpose, which is to provide an increased capability for the maintenance of health and the management of disease and thus be more effective and satisfying to the needs of medicine.

It is my conviction that if such laudable ends are to be achieved, there must be some satisfaction of the continuing need for serious reexamination of the participant's roles in a very complex research undertaking—the federal agencies, the scientists, and their institutions and resources—as well as of the socioeconomic environment within which the system operates. I would emphasize that such an examination should not be yet another conventional study of the biomedical field. The number of those in the past make quite obvious the need for some type of continuing study of this national activity, one that recognizes political reality but is not dominated by political concerns; that has a keen perception of societal needs, but only as a part of the backdrop against which programs must evolve; and that is not dominated by the academics, yet has a clear perception of their needs and capabilities.

What I have in mind is the likely need for establishment of a continuing audit, as untrammeled as possible from bias, and certainly not directly responsible to those who are major supporters of science, those who directly utilize science, or indeed those of society itself that benefit. I think this can be done if several of the great foundations can be made to appreciate the complexity, the urgency, and the importance of the problem enough for some of them to undertake such a continuing study during the coming decade.

The need becomes imperative if one reviews very briefly what has happened within the biomedical sciences during the past fifty years. In 1929, science and biomedicine had a narrow base, and there were few professional scientists. Biomedical research was a part-time avocation of some intelligent, interested people, many of whom had little formal training. Many studies were perforce undertaken in the absence of a broad background of biology, which we now know is important to understand if we are to comprehend the phenomena of disease. Yet the institutionalization of biomedical science, such as it was in 1929, was really the fruit of some three decades of progressive developments, starting with a few institutions at the turn of the century, such as the universities of Wisconsin, Michigan, Harvard, Johns Hopkins, and Pennsylvania.

By and large, these institutions, together with the Rockefeller Institute for Medical Research, contained the bulk of our scientific capital at the end of the last century. Yet by 1929 there was a modest but broadly diversified system of medical education, operating at relatively low cost, having been developed from the few institutions noted here that were in operation at the turn of the century, and stimulated by a very critical report by Abraham Flexner in 1910 on the deficiencies in American medical education, a will on the part of many institutions to improve, and a number of private foundations and private donors who were willing to foot the bill. Certainly a good start had been made.

By contrast, we now have a broadly diversified science base, generally characterized by excellence and utilized by a substantial number of highly trained professional scientists who are continuously productive. But this system, lest we become too enthusiastic, has its problems. The program of research and its related education programs are housed in institutions that are highly unstable, with little capability for managing their own affairs, particularly against a rapidly increasing inflation. They have developed an absolute dependency on the actions of a number of federal agencies that bear directly on their complex activities. They are characterized by a contraction in stable career opportunities and a categorical system of research support that was essential to the Public Health Service to meet its own obligations in the postwar initiation of its programs. The support of research at the National Institutes of Health (NIH) along categorical lines effectively emphasized the growing importance of chronic illness at mid-century. But such a setting is less able to provide a base as the medical sciences, in all their complexity, must probe deeper and deeper in fields of fundamental biology. The nature and operation of these biological systems warrant broad support; yet at a time of lower budgets and expanding needs for medical research in general, and with a continuing drive for research in applied areas, the needs of science have long outstripped the general support programs that provide for the biological programs within the present organization of NIH.

Thus there would appear to be basic deficiencies in the support system itself. And since it is primarily a federal system, and primarily centered in NIH, the formulation of budget within the social setting of the Congress determines the strategy of approach to the problems, and implementation of the programs may have grave defects. These are not simple problems. The utility and wisdom of a categorical program must be reexamined in the light of shifting needs and their satisfaction in both the applied and developmental areas, as well as in the formalized mix of the two. I'm quite certain that a large portion of NIH continues to be guided by categorical needs, but I think this must be suitably balanced by a less categorical approach to a major portion of the scientific opportunities that exist today.

Recognition of the problem is not difficult. The catchword now is *basic* science, although I'm not quite sure what basic science is. Those of the Cancer Institute will say that today the institute is supporting more basic science than NIH as a whole supported ten years ago. If that is true, I think it's a great tragedy. I don't believe that such basic science as it does support is emotionally and scientifically best suited to be a part of an urgent effort to bring the fruits of science to bear on a set of very practical problems. I would prefer to see such a program operating within the physical, chemical, and mathematical mix that is obtained in the basic scientific laboratory rather than within the framework of an emotional drive that derives its support from the very practical and worthwhile objectives of the Cancer Institute. These thoughts may seem to be mere quibbling, minor things—of bureaucratic importance, perhaps, but hardly of scientific importance. But I'm convinced that as we raise our young scientists in the generations to come, we do them no good by exposing them to the social urgencies of medicine that have little expression in their own day-to-day work.

It would be wise at this point to consider, for example, a re-engineering of institutional research grants and a system of institution-based research fellowships that might stabilize the university biomedical environment. The push for knowledge must find some reasonably stable mechanism within the university centers for their core activities, rather than continuing to depend on the present multitude of individual grant and contract programs. I'm convinced that our programs could be more productive and more satisfying than they are today. These mechanics were useful in program formulation and execution in the earlier days, at lower budget levels. A fresh look is not only desirable but essential.

Looking to the future, in an assessment of what may be considered to be an adequate value (or a floor, a ceiling, or both) for research in the biomedical sciences, one must also consider methods of funding that tie the research expenditure to the purchasing power of the dollar. Estimates for the future must also provide a set of parameters that can serve as guides to the continuing evaluation of the changing substance of the research program and the level of manpower and facilities that are desirable. These estimates must also afford some measure of stability for the institutions that house the process. Such considerations are difficult, if not impossible, to include in the annually recurring budget cycle.

The impact of socially oriented groups on the biomedical research budget of NIH has gotten out of hand. The topic of societal needs as related to the allocation of resources cannot be simply introduced by a series of questions that relate to the socioeconomic impact of serious disease and the elements of suitable counterprograms in research, in education, and in the medical service systems. When one considers societal needs in a more general fashion, it is apparent that the needs and programs concerned with health are broader than those of medicine. In this light, one should consider the price the nation is now paying for the assortment of activities that relate to health, and what proportion such a health cost has in the aggregate costs of all people-related expenditures.

It is clear that there is little summary data that bear on such a problem, and there is difficulty in determining what is to be included in the various cost centers. The calculus contains many very broad considerations that are not conventionally presented as solvable problems, at least as reflected in the federal budget. But the very complexity of the problem should encourage the establishment of some approximations that can serve as general guides in program development, and, of course, in resource allocation. It is reasonable to conclude, for purposes of our present planning, that a point in our nation's development has been reached where in real income it is at a "no growth" stage—and that this has happened when there remains a number of broad and important unmet social needs, which are to be found in such areas as general education, housing, and income maintenance, as well as in health. In such a view, any increase in real support for the complex of research, education, and medical services must come at the expense of other activities, and there will be fierce competition for each such dollar gained or lost.

In consequence, it becomes of paramount importance for medicine to examine its national expenditures and decide in association with the executive branch and Congress how its present funding can be allocated across, and within, each of the three elements of research, education, and service, and what the federal role should be in the partial support of each activity.

It would appear important, as a matter of federal policy, to secure for the biomedical sciences a strong base in the universities and their related professional schools as an essential for a strong national effort. Although many elements of such a base were provided for in the late 1950s and early 1960s, the goal itself was never simply, clearly, and explicitly enunciated as an essential part of a desirable national policy. Some federal intent was clear in the statements of appropriation and legislative committees and those of several secretaries of HEW and Presidents. But still, there is nowhere to be found a freestanding statement of federal policy made by well-constituted authority.

The arguments that favor the need for an adequate and stable academic base are many. These academic institutions and their related enterprises provide the nation on a continuing basis with the general science grounding for a reasonable health program. They provide the fundamental training for all scientists—federal, industrial, and academic alike—and the related professionals of the medical and biomedical establishment, and the continuing education of this establishment. They also provide the institutionalization of a major portion of the biomedical research and development programs though there is a suitable, nonduplicative sharing of this responsibility with the industrial and federal segments of science.

It should not have to be argued in detail that there is a need for the continued support of academically oriented federal programs at realistic levels. One can only conclude that research, education, and specialized training in the biomedical fields are essential for the nation's health and its health care systems, and that the biomedical sciences in place at academic institutions constitute an important and essential part of the more general medical establishment.

It is less simple to define, within the academic and related institutions, the elements that are essential and of special concern to the federal establishment. It is clear that the size and character of the science base and the amount of stability required for an effective operation are only amenable to estimates based on informed judgments, and these may vary widely.

Nonetheless, a beginning can be made by accepting the view that any broad and essential part of a complex academic endeavor requires some measure of internal stability for its own effective operation. The academic endeavor should include:

1.   The major research programs of an institution

2. The cadre of scientists and educators essential for the satisfaction of the institutional mission
3. The institutional framework and mechanisms essential for effective interaction among the programs of research, education, and service
4. Those elements that provide for participation in the renewal of the system, the effective operation of which tends toward its own obsolescence

The basic legislation that provides the authorizations for the diversified programs of the NIH does not in addition explicitly provide for each of these essential needs, and it is unlikely that it ever will. It is for these reasons that the NIH fostered the view that only a portion of such a set of needs should be satisfied by the support of research, training, and related resources within the categorical structure of the NIH. But much can be accomplished with the grant-in-aid as the major instrument. This requires careful attention to the terms and conditions of the grant and its renewal. The NIH has had broad authority to do these things and also to develop programs that, when properly administered, satisfy an essential need of categorical programs and yet additionally, and quite directly, contribute stability to an institution as a by-product.

But it would be a distortion of the NIH mission were it to attempt to satisfy the total needs of the concerned institutions. Within the present systems of support, the problem of institutional instability emerges acutely when institutions have more or less complete dependence for their integrity upon research-related support, and at the same time the realities of the academic situation clearly indicate that the mission of the institution is a broad mix of coupled responsibilities in research, instruction, and service.

The terms and conditions of support for research-dependent functions have been continuously adjusted in the development of the NIH so that the derivative programs are generally supportive of the broader purposes of an institution. But they are less effective in the aggregate now than heretofore, due to general shortage of funds and selective cuts in programs. It is interesting, in these regards, that many costly programs of the National Science Foundation are directed toward attempts to couple new information to societal need; yet in the case of the biomedical sciences, where such an effective coupling mechanism already exists—that is, in the medical center—there is little concern for the continuing maintenance of these centers as a stable base for a number of essential scientific and educational activities of profound national concern.

The institutions of concern here are the universities, the medical centers, research-oriented hospitals, research institutes, and industry. Let us make the practical problem somewhat simpler by pointing out that industry, though it now maintains a broadly diversified research program, has come to grips with its problems of a need for stability and continuity of purpose. It now only requires reasonable management and intelligent control of its activities by the federal establishment. Given these and a separate source of high-quality young scientists, it can adjust its research and development activities to its goals within an industrial structure based on a reasonable profit return.

But the academic environments have no such tie to stability. Quite apart from large appropriations for research and from profound uncertainties in the manpower and educational fields, the funds available for research itself are quite unstable.

As the result of such evidence of inconstant purpose, the biomedical sciences, though still productive, are in a difficult position in the longer view. Further, good programs always require a fair measure of freedom of action in their execution, and the need for this increases as fiscal constraints are imposed. Meanwhile, there is too little concern on the part of scientists with the things that determine the integrity of the federal programs and their academic base and perhaps too much concern with the funding of activities within their own areas of interest.

THE EXPANDING BASE OF SCIENTIFIC KNOWLEDGE

David A. Hamburg, M.D.
President, Institute of Medicine

We were not much oriented to the significance of fundamental scientific investigation in this country until World War II, and nothing in our history brought home so vividly the lesson of the practicality of basic research as the work in atomic physics that led to all the subsequent developments in the war. It was a painful but important lesson for us to absorb, not only in physics but in every field of science—that there is nothing so practical as a good theory, and that fundamental investigation might have many largely unforeseeable practical consequences. However, in ensuing decades we tended a bit to lose sight of the fact that that arrow goes both ways between basic research and clinical observation. It was easy to forget, for example, that the landmark discovery that DNA is a genetic material grew out of Avery's interests in pneumonia. Very messy clinical problems of pneumonia led him to the famous pneumococcal transformation experiments that elucidated the critical role of DNA as a genetic material. So it is a continuing interplay, not just a flow, from basic science to clinical application.

We have to adjust science policy to new conditions as circumstances change, and the linkage of clinical investigation and basic research has been one of the very important contributions of the National Institutes of Health, whose work has built respect and credibility for NIH as an institution, and indeed for American health sciences altogether. I would say today that NIH has truly a worldwide eminence. I was impressed, for example, when we went to China in June 1979 to negotiate a health science agreement, with the extent to which they not only had enormous respect for NIH but knew in considerable detail about its nature and functions. And that has been my experience in all parts of the world, not only in the highly industrialized countries where you'd expect such knowledge. In my judgment, the respect for American science in general and health science in particular is potentially one of our bulwarks in today's world, where so many prejudicial stereotypes about America exist. This is an area of great strength, and I'm inclined to think that in general public policy we have not sufficiently developed and utilized the strength that is embedded in that enormous respect. I would say it was always Dr. Shannon's characteristic that he was restlessly pressing at the frontiers of knowledge; he had an openness to new scientific opportunities and their possible linkages to health and disease, and one such area in which I've benefited personally was his early appreciation of the emerging potentiality of neurobiology. I naturally tend to take as a base line my own point of entry into clinical psychiatry and basic research on behavioral biology, three decades ago.

What a difference three decades can make! How very much more we have come to understand the brain and the rest of the nervous system than we had anticipated would be possible in those days, and that progress has been accelerated by this continuing interplay between research and clinical investigation. For instance, clinical observations on the severe depressions, and also hypertension, have a lot to do with progress in understanding the nature of the nervous system. Research on brain function has really been stimulated by drug treatment—mostly empirically derived—for mental, neurological, and cardiovascular disorders, and as some even modest advances came to be verified, then people wondered about the mechanism of action of the drugs that affect the brain. That led to a deeper examination of the way the human brain works and brought into the field a whole generation of young investigators who are fascinated with its awesome complexity—one of the great frontiers that is just now emerging in its full potentiality. If one looks ahead for the remainder of this century, it's got to be one of the principal areas of advance in all of science, not only in the life sciences.

The human brain is composed of about 10 billion nerve cells of incredible complexity. The long nerve-cell processes, the axons, conduct electrical impulses; the axons connect to other neurons in very elaborate circuitry; one axon does not actually touch the next one but is separated by a cleft, and the connections between those are chemical. When a neuron fires, it releases a neurotransmitter or neuroregulator that diffuses across the gap and attaches to a receptor on the second neuron, and there that activates a mechanism that may stimulate, inhibit, or modify the firing of the next neuron. Several neurons, some stimulating, some inhibiting, are connected to one neuron by some of these neurotransmitters. So the molecules that serve as neurotransmitters, or that modify that transaction, the neuroregulators, have come to be enormously interesting, and the drugs that affect the brain act chiefly by influencing these neurotransmitters and neuroregulators. The transmission of information in the brain—that is to say, how cells in the brain talk to each other, and in addition how cells in the brain talk to the rest of the body and regulate the functions of the various systems in the body—is certainly one of the cutting edges in the health sciences at the present time.

Transmitters have been identified and in the past few years have come to be called conventional transmitters. Two decades ago we barely had a clue about any transmitter, and yet now we have a dozen that are already called conventional. They are differentially distributed, and that differential distribution in the brain has some relationship to their functional activity. They are very heavily concentrated in circuits that control the endocrine, the autonomic, and the cardiovascular systems, but they are also linked to memory appraisal and motivation and emotional responses. What is so fascinating, therefore, is that we are not only learning something about the brain functions that mediate our essential psychological processes but also about the way in which the brain exercises controls over functions throughout the body.

In the past few years, a whole new class of neuroregulators has emerged, the neuropeptides, which have an action not in milliseconds, like the conventional transmitters, but in minutes or even hours, a totally unanticipated development. They appear, so to say, to sit on the receptor for a long period of time and modulate the flow of information in the brain, evidently a kind of fine tuning or coordination of the coordinators—that is, of the two great coordinating systems of the body, the central nervous system and the endocrine system. Investigators identified a few peptides that are secreted in the brain and pass from the brain to the anterior pituitary and thence to every cell and tissue in the body. So we get a very specific connection between molecular biology and organism biology, and a tying together of the organism, because that organism is more than a bag of molecules; the parts have to work together. The brilliant elucidation of the components of the organism, the molecular and cellular levels, is, I suppose, the greatest single advance in the life sciences, perhaps in any sciences, in the past two decades. Those components must work together or we will not have a functioning, adaptable, viable organism.

These neurotransmitters, which are mostly either monoamines or acids, and the neuropeptides, which are slightly more complex molecules, affect a number of functions that are of enormous interest in medicine and to the public at large. They not only influence a number of cardiovascular and gastrointestinal functions, but also functions like sexual behavior, alertness, the relief of pain, sense of well-being, release of distress, promotion of sleep, control of appetite, and various aspects of learning and memory. So in this field, as in some others like immunology and genetics, we are talking about enormous opportunities for medical practice of the future.

There are a number of benefits already apparent from the new neurobehavioral biology. For example, the phenothiazines for schizophrenia, lithium for depressive disorders, tricyclic antidepressants, beta blockers in certain aspects of cardiovascular disease, and the benzodiazopines in anxiety. Yet in order to be realistic about these advances we have to recognize that we've already seen problems with them that are generic in character and that we can expect to see ramified, and probably amplified, in the decades ahead. One of these is excessive public expectations. Another is a tendency of physicians to overprescribe, and still another is the emergence of long-term side effects that a certain number of patients get when treated with phenothiazines. Yet another is that long-acting metabolites may accumulate and interact with alcohol or other drugs that affect the brain, in such way as to impair motor performance— for example, driving a car.

So there are complications in this powerful array of new brain-active medications, and we can expect, in principle, that the same will be true of the even more powerful set that will emerge in the next decade or so. When you're talking about medications that affect, say, sexual behavior, sleep, the release of emotional stress, or pain, you can expect some leakage out of the medical system into a kind of street ecology. You can expect the establishment of neighborhood laboratories, because there will be a very high incentive to have these drugs readily available, and much of the chemistry is not all that arcane. So there are problems connected with this enormously growing power that we have for therapeutic and preventive interventions. For medical practice, I think a critical element is to get adequate research data, readily available, and to facilitate the ability of physicians and other practitioners to keep up with new developments.

I've gone into this exploding line of inquiry—neurobiology and its clinical implications—to illustrate our increasing power in health care, which I think will enlarge greatly over the next two or three decades. Like all power, it may be used for better or for worse; perhaps it's realistic to say both for better and for worse. How can we use it wisely? Neither plausibility nor authority can substitute for evidence, and thus the responsibility of health research to generate evidence is greater now than before.

I want to emphasize a concept that I think is critical, because I think it's an area in which health insurers, both public and private, must become more deeply involved. That is to view the health sciences as a chain, a long chain, each link of which must be strong if the whole chain is to bear the full weight of improving health over the years to come. This chain links the quest for basic information on the nature of living organisms, including the human organism, to demonstrably useful interventions in the prevention, diagnosis, and treatment of disease. It's not enough to have the fundamental knowledge generate insights; the way in which those insights relate to our patients and to the public remains also to be ascertained by scientific means.

Therefore, in the next couple of decades we will have to complete this spectrum of health research, and that includes several major components. One is the fostering of basic inquiry, about which I need say no more, and another is scanning that knowledge base for promising, health-relevant applications. I say promising because some will work out, and some won't, but those that are promising need to be examined and fostered very carefully. A third component is analyzing the burdens of illness in the population in relation to scientific opportunity, because science policy always ends up being some kind of interaction between these problems and the opportunities. Finally, we must build the practice of the health professions on a solid, scientific base to ensure that the knowledge base of health care will develop strongly in the years to come. This last effort will involve research on the benefits, risks, and costs of diagnostic, therapeutic, and preventive interventions, as well as research on the organization, financing, and delivery of health services. Public and private health insurers will, I think, increasingly feel the need for more dependable information on these questions of health care, and there must be active support for such health care research so that we may ascertain what we're actually doing to obtain better results from the fruits of basic discovery.

To complete the task of building a health sciences chain strong in all its links is a formidable enterprise that goes far beyond any single institution. I'm not advocating that this task should be taken on by NIH alone: it is one for society as a whole. To complete that chain will require ingenuity, innovation, and persistence, not only in science itself but in appropriate institutional arrangements of government, universities, industry, and the professions to foster the sciences in all their complexity. This task will require a longer range time scale and a broader view than we have been accustomed to in the past. It will require orderly means for preserving what is best in our research traditions and for stimulating change where the burdens are heavy and emerging opportunities may be perceived.

THE SHANNON LEGACY AND MEDICAL RESEARCH TODAY

Donald S. Fredrickson, M.D.
Director, National Institutes of Health

Any doubt that this is America's century in medicine will surely be dispelled when its history is written. This is largely attributable to the quality of the medical science that has
developed in this country since the century opened. Early
benchmarks on that ascending curve would surely include the
formation of a clinical research unit at Johns Hopkins in about
1900—the first such unit that I know of anywhere. Others
would be the opening of the Rockefeller Hospital in 1910, aug-
menting the already thriving Institute for Medical Research;
and, at about the same time, the influence of American clinical
research in Great Britain. Still another important development was the transformation and expansion of the present National Institutes of Health (NIH) out of what had been a small
in-house laboratory for the Public Health Service. Many have
contributed to that latter achievement; probably no single figure stands out more prominently than James A. Shannon.

In 1968 Dr. Shannon retired from another position, this time
as the eighth director of NIH. His tenure of thirteen years was
the longest in the history of that demanding position. When, in
1975, I succeeded him in this chair, the NIH he had left and
the NIH I would now head were not so different. But the world
in which it operated had changed greatly in seven years. The
end of the 1960s had seen the trial and torment of elite institutions of all kinds, and science was not spared. The ethical
frames in which we had to perform were shifting. There was a
prescriptive element to the political economy surrounding
medicine and its scientific base. A major source of anxiety was
the rate of rise in the cost of health care, and some felt certain
that science must be partly to blame.

There was, too, a sudden expansion in the power of experi-
mental biology, which gave rise to anxieties of another kind. I
began to engage in some problems that Jim Shannon would

have found strongly antitraditional. For one, I acquired the task of promulgating guidelines for the conduct of genetic engineering in terms of the techniques for using recombinant DNA. About 40 percent of my time in my first two years was devoted to coping with the confrontation between some anxious critics and a concerned but angry segment of the scientific community. Each was suspicious of the other, and yet they were trying to draw together—to close the gap of perception between the laity and the scientists and among many scientists themselves.

I also surveyed worriedly the boundaries of NIH, lines whose shape also fixed the azimuth of medical science in America. I was concerned, particularly, with what was, and what was not, appropriate for an organization whose objectivity was crucial and whose resources, although great, were always less than the sum of congressional expectations for scientific solutions. We had to seize some appropriate roles in resolving the suspicions and social problems that had sprung from modern biomedical technology. We had to restore confidence in the ability of our science to address practical problems. As one response, we began the technology assessment exercises—the "searches for consensus," carefully programmed analyses of the state of the art that have recently made NIH much more of a household word to physicians than heretofore.

Third, we engaged in activities that I think Jim Shannon would also have viewed with bemusement. We have sat for many hours with all the sister agencies of the Public Health Service in an ecumenical effort to get the health sciences in the Department of Health and Human Services to recognize certain common principles for federal funding in the future. We looked at questions that have become increasingly nagging over three or four years. None of the cries is more demanding than those of the regulatory agencies seeking instant knowledge to help them to meet their mandates for regulation. In addition, there are the rising questions of whether we can improve and expand health services research and perform more clinical trials to refine better the substance of medical practice today and to assist in setting some limits to the growth of its cost. Such health research planning—the straining for a global perspective—has not been all comfortable. Yet we have begun to address the complementarity of the agencies in ways that both improve the federal presence in health as well as leave its research arm free of activities inappropriate for medical science.

There are signs of progress. The new National Center for Health Care Technology, an HHS institution, will take up some of the most value-laden questions about new and old inventions that make up the fabric of health care. NIH can be properly concerned with only the technical and scientific questions here.

We are approaching a point in the evolution of NIH guidelines for DNA research that establishes them as the primary standard for the world, and in ways that now see the technology expanding and flourishing without excessive regulation and cumbersome statutory restriction.

In fostering certain special programs that relate us to the regulatory agencies, like the National Toxicology Program, we have gainsaid a great deal of the criticism that we were indifferent to the practical needs of the regulatory agencies. Thus we can enhance their search for standards, join them to the cutting edge of scientific advance, and avoid our participating directly in regulatory activities.

I think, too, that we are beginning to see the emergence of several agencies, notably the Center for Disease Control in the Public Health Service, with a stronger role in health promotion, again making it possible for the boundaries of NIH to be drawn in such a way that we can avoid placing our objectivity in peril by excessive peddling of the inventions emerging from science.

To me, these were the most important tasks of the last five years—crucial hurdles to mount in order that we might get on to some of the other issues raised by Dr. Shannon. There is no question in my mind that the power of biological and medical science today is greater than it was when I came to NIH. For example, there is the extraordinary capability that we now have in molecular biology. I am sure that it will eventually be possible to make in bacteria virtually any product of human genes. This will create cheaper and purer supplies of hormones, other biologicals, and monovalent vaccines against a whole variety of agents. We may even be able to control the instability of the influenza virus in a practical way to make better live vaccines. There is no foreseeable limit to the future of medical science in better serving the preventive and curative practices in American medicine.

Clinical trials will continue. They impose a special burden, but our ability to perform them well certainly reflects the developments that occurred when Jim Shannon was trustee of the nation's medical research apparatus.

I think we have now begun to cope with another major problem—stabilization of the support for science in this country. And I speak not only of fundamental science, but of clinical science as well. With the growth of NIH, a social contract came into being in America. It is not derived from natural law, but from a sense of opportunity for scientists and the public to do a job together in using human creativity in the most humane and useful ways. We must find in the 1980s ways to insure the exceedingly close relationship between fundamental work in the life sciences and the constant movement of the findings toward practical use in society. The basic and the applied efforts do lie at opposite ends of a spectrum, and their social support and economic underpinning do derive, as Dr. Shannon has pointed out, from different sentiments. Yet, if I argue that the isolation of basic from applied research would split the continuum of medical science, it is not to deny serious problems within the educational institutions where most of the research goes on. Furthermore, it is apparent that the universities and the government do not understand each other well. Charges that regulations and procedures are stifling research, on the one hand, and of fraud and lack of accountability for public money, on the other, are symptoms of disorder for which simple prescriptions are not available. Speaking for the NIH of Dr. Shannon and his successors, I know that we shall commit much of our time and energies in the coming year to understanding and relieving some of the distress that he perceives.

IV INVITED ADDRESSES

THE ROLE OF THE THIRD SECTOR IN A VOLUNTARY SOCIETY

Kingman Brewster, Jr.
U.S. Ambassador to the United Kingdom

In institutional terms, a birthday is a milestone that prompts reflection on the purpose that gave it birth and rededication to that purpose for the uncounted years ahead. It is my pretentious assignment to consider not the original purpose, the fifty years of accomplishment, or the prospect of Blue Cross and Blue Shield. Walter McNerney was irresponsible enough to ask me to address our society, our nation; where it came from, where it has been, where it is going. I was irresponsible enough to accept.

In thinking about our colonial origins, I am put in mind of a *New Yorker* cartoon in which two pilgrim fathers leaning on the taffrail of the Mayflower are in conversation. One turns to the other and says, "Religious freedom is my immediate goal, but my long-range plan is to go into real estate." So it has been, down the generations of immigration to America. Hope for material betterment was part of the promise. But even deeper was, and is, the hope that in the New World you stood a chance of being your own man. To worship according to your own faith without fear of persecution. To think and express your own thoughts without fear of prosecution. To criticize and oppose authority without fear of retribution. To do your own thing in your own way, taking the risk of the marketplace without having to ask anyone's approval in advance.

I have tried to find a word or a phrase that captures the spirit of the American purpose, the American adventure. The best I have been able to do is to call it an unending struggle to create and to perpetuate and to perfect a "voluntary society."

Our first enemy was a coercive government, high-handed, at worst; at best, unrepresentative and unresponsive to its colonial subjects. It was because we felt entitled to the "rights of Englishmen" that we declared our independence from the Crown.

The Declaration spelled out the infringements that provoked our exasperation. However, we declared our rights in the name of all human beings, who by birthright were entitled to life, liberty, and the pursuit of happiness.

When we came to frame a constitution for the government of our new country, we were determined to constrain the powers of government so that a new tyranny would not arise to replace the old.

If life was to be as voluntary as possible for the citizen, the powers of central government should be distributed among co-equal branches, subject to redress and review if limits on authority should be transgressed either at the expense of the citizen or at the expense of state and local self-determination. The union itself was threatened by differences about the legality of human slavery. A bloody Civil War saved the union and resulted in further limits on state as well as federal ability to deprive any citizen of the equal protection of the laws.

Under both the First and Fourteenth Amendments, civil rights and liberties were expanded by judicial interpretation and legislation. Society was by law made more voluntary for the unpopular and for every racial minority.

Life can be made involuntary, liberty frustrated, and the pursuit of happiness denied not only by coercive government, but also by economic and social circumstance. For the first 150 years of our history, this was not a primary direct concern of government.

Hope for a new life, a fresh start, a better prospect for one's children if not oneself, was sustained by the promise of the frontier. Financial and corporate ingenuity devised ways of assembling capital to make the most of the resources of a vast, rich continent. New tools, new processes, new sources of energy, new techniques of organization achieved a pace of economic growth that kept opportunity alive, even as the physical frontier reached its continental limits.

The same financial and corporate ingenuity that made this taming of the continent possible also brought forth its own threat to the voluntary society. It took the form of trusts and combinations with power to coerce shippers, suppress competition, and exploit customers. When the railroads had all long-distance haulage to themselves, the Interstate Commerce Act was passed to protect the shippers. When the oil, tobacco, and sugar trusts became private governments with no limits on their power to exploit suppliers, competitors and customers, the Sherman Antitrust Act was passed. Later it was given vigor by Theodore Roosevelt's trustbusting. The regulatory state, under the banner of Woodrow Wilson's "New Freedom," gave some assurance that government would take on the responsibility for keeping society as voluntary as possible despite the growth of private power. The tradition of skepticism of government bigness, which was at the roots of our constitutional design, found counterpart in the new anti–Wall Street populism. As attorney Louis Brandeis is reported to have said to the court when arguing against one of the railroad combines: "Your honor, if the Good Lord meant us to have such large organizations, he would have given us the brains to run them."

It was not until the New Deal, brought on by the Great Depression, however, that government assumed a pervasive responsibility for dealing directly with economic and social challenges to the voluntary society. Farmers who sold in a highly competitive market and had to buy in a much less competitive market were given huge subsidies and were rewarded for producing less under the AAA. In order to trim the balance of bargaining power, labor's right to organize was encouraged by the Wagner Act. For a brief while, all of industry was organized into a corporate state under the NRA. For those who were still left out of productive employment, the WPA, then the PWA and the CCC were created. The war superseded them all. Then inflation became the challenge. It was kept under control by forced savings and legally imposed wage and price ceilings.

The "Fair Deal," and later the "New Frontier" and the "Great Society," made it clear that forevermore a representative government could not evade its responsibility for maintaining the level of national economic activity. Government took on the job of protecting the citizen against the new enemy of a voluntary society—loss of economic hope.

The challenges of trying to prevent government from interfering with the voluntary life of the citizen and of using government to protect the citizen against economic hopelessness are still with us. Partisan rhetoric tends in an election year to try to make us believe that we must choose between the two. If we are to be true to the vision of a society that is as voluntary as possible for all its citizens, we must continue to try to have it both ways: limited government and widespread economic opportunity. Happily—since I don't have one—this is not the place to prescribe a solution. But in passing let me mention three matters that seem to me badly in need of more attention than they now receive:

First, because more and more of what we do is dependent upon government support, we must find some way to bring what I would call the "money license" under a rule of law. When the government has a power of life or death over a firm because of government subsidies, loans, guarantees, or contracts, the fairness of its decisions should be no less subject to judicial review than administrative regulations are.

Second, government has become increasingly the biggest influence on how much is spent on consumption and how much is saved for long-term investment. We must find some way of offsetting the tendency of officeholders elected for a short term to favor consumption "now" at the expense of investment or conservation that won't pay out in jobs or goods until some remote "then," well beyond the next election.

Third, government now has the power and the need to contract economic activity in order to prevent it from being evaporated in inflation. We must devise some way of assuring that the burden of contraction falls on those most able to bear it, not primarily on those on the bottom rungs of the social and economic ladder—those deprived of jobs.

These are today's problems, not only for the United States but for the rest of the industrialized, more or less democratic, world. I am sure we shall solve them.

There is another threat to the voluntary society, however, that seems to be just around the corner of the microprocessed society. Bigness is here to stay—in business, in government, in labor organizations. Technology has made manageable organizations of scope and complexity that would have defied the day of the quill pen, the telegraph boy on a bicycle, and the telephone you rang with a crank. Bigness demands the development of routines susceptible to computerization, both for direction and for accountability. With complex routines comes specialization at higher and higher levels of complexity, coded by increasingly mystifying equations, jargon, and acronyms. Whether or not, in Brandeis' phrase, the Good Lord intended us to have such large organizations, we have, in a sense, developed the brains to run them, provided we have the judgment to guide the mechanized brains that the computer and microchip give us.

Of course, the goods and services made possible by these miracles are a fantastic boon. But what does it all portend for the voluntary society? What happens to individual identity? What happens to the satisfaction of making a constructive impact on the lives of others? What happens to personal purpose?

I ask you to take an inward look. All of us spend part of our time, spend a large part of our energy, and consume an enormous amount of our worry reserve on some activity or cause or organization that is not for profit and not for votes. It may be an orchestra or gallery; it may be a community service; it may be the board of a library, a hospital, or a recreation center, a school or a college. As the processes of big business and big government do, increasingly specialized professions make it increasingly hard to discern one's vocational impact on the total situation or on any other human being, I suggest that it is the voluntary sector of community life that becomes more and more important.

It rekindles my faith in the dispersion of social, economic, and political power. We horse-and-buggy federalists may have to surrender much of home rule and states' rights to the necessities of governing an interdependent continent. We populist trustbusters may have to lie down and be flattened by the conglomerations of capital that modern finance, supply, production, and distribution on an international scale require. A vital and dispersed voluntary sector, however, may provide the purpose and identity that can so easily be squeezed out by the growing impersonal bigness of the public and private sectors.

Most voluntary organizations arise from a shared sense of community needs. They are intensely local. They provide the satisfaction of being able to see and touch and feel the impact of what you do on the people you are trying to help. Even if the organizations are as complex as hospitals or universities, still they tend to be local establishments—more like the neighborhood store than the chain store supermarket.

But not only are most nonprofit organizations local, they are quite autonomous in their self-government. It may be, and often is, true that responsible offices and directorships, even commodores of yacht clubs, and certainly so-called voluntary fund-raisers, have to be conscripted by fraud, duress, and arm twisting. Nevertheless, they are not imposed by some absentee public or private authority.

The microprocessor and the computer printout may impose, in the name of managerial efficiency, a sameness on the fingers and toes of a massive organization. The voluntary sector will by its local nature sustain the richness that variety permits. Such variety is inevitable as long as the activity, organization, and institution are a reflection of the needs and idiosyncrasies and traditions of a local community, not the fine print of some federal regulation or corporate directive.

Because of the inevitability of bigness in the profitmaking and the vote-seeking sectors, I would assert that the voluntary sector is an important element in a purposeful voluntary life. This is significant in terms of a society as well as in terms of the individual. The variety and pluralism of private, nonprofit activity are perhaps most important in the area of private philanthropic support of scholarship, research, and new ideas generally. If a new idea could not shop around the voluntary sector for support, if its chances of being given a fair try depended upon the echelons of a single bureaucracy, the likelihood of the truly novel, far-out approach gaining support would be greatly diminished. Especially if the new approach challenges the way of doing things that the bureaucracy has already invested in, it will not be welcome. Philanthropists are not a notoriously bold lot; but they are a healthy antidote to the risklessness that is too likely to permeate an entrenched, impersonal bureaucracy. For the same reason, tens of hundreds of foundations and individual philanthropists are far better than any one alone.

This leads to the third aspect of the voluntary sector—over and above its outlet for individual purpose and its capacity to sustain the variety of centers of support on which intellectual innovation depends. What I have in mind might be called the "private yardstick."

When I was awakening to public matters in the 1930s, there was a great deal of controversy surrounding the proposal for a Tennessee Valley Authority. Its ultimate justification was to provide a public yardstick by which to measure the efficiency, as well as the fairness, of the rates of privately owned electric utilities. Now it seems to me the shoe is on the other foot, not in electric power generation, but in a host of activities and services that have become predominantly governmental responsibilities. In health, education, and welfare, for example, to take the range of public responsibilities elevated to cabinet status by President Eisenhower (not, be it noted, under any hyperbolic slogans such as New Deal, Fair Deal, New Frontier, or Great Society), the private yardstick of the voluntary sector is of crucial importance if public performance is to be held to a high standard.

The one I know best is higher education. The "market share" of the private institutions has steadily shrunk. Not only in share but in quality, the great state universities, even in the East (long since in the Midwest and Far West) have evolved far beyond the "aggies" of my youth. They have become first-rate centers of research, scholarship, and education in the liberal arts and learned professions, as well as in agriculture and the mechanical arts, which had given them life under the Land Grant Act. The best of the state institutions have been the equal of, if not superior to, the strongest of the older private universities. Nevertheless, there is not a state university president or chancellor who has not been grateful for the tradition of self-government, independence, and academic freedom of his private competitors. These values are bound to be much more vulnerable in a university dependent upon a state legislature than in a privately supported institution. The tradition of private trusteeship not only keeps the faculty from embezzling the funds, it also keeps donors from trying to dictate the direction of learning. Indeed, I know of one case where a state university president took along a trustee of a private university to appear before a legislative budget committee to make the point that inadequate support or improper interference with faculty freedom would permit the visitor's institution to abduct the best of the local faculty.

In the field of higher education, it seems to me essential to have some institutions that are not beholden to either the marketplace or the ballot box. Popularity, either in the sense of sales or in the sense of votes, cannot be the test of truth. If the quest for a better explanation of things were to be distorted by fear of disfavor or desire for favor, neither research nor instruction would retain their credibility. Academic credibility derives from a search for, and an expression of, truth guided only by the dictates of a conscientious intellect. It is not surprising, therefore, that the vitality of American higher education is the envy of the world, since it has, in its origin and in its evolution, been led and leavened by largely self-determined faculties, protected by private trustees, nurtured by accumulated private gifts and endowments. Donors, by and large, have not sought to usurp the faculty's responsibility for collective direction of academic affairs and have not sought to infringe the individual scholar's academic freedom. Each of us can think of a public-school system that has benefited from self-conscious comparison with its private rivals, or public-health facilities whose standards are set by comparing them with those of private institutions. Even public architectural standards can be influenced by the boldness of the nonprofit sector, although not all can do as well as J. Irwin Miller has in Columbus, Indiana. The private yardstick does make a difference.

I would submit that there are some activities that would be quite stultified if they had to rely solely on either the vote-seeking or the profitmaking motivation. I have mentioned education already. Another is the creative and performing arts. Also, there is health care.

In the area of the creative and performing arts, the vitality of painting, sculpture, drama, and music in America has been sustained largely by community, foundation, and individual private support. Many of the greatest galleries and museums, symphony orchestras, and opera and repertory companies have very largely been supported by private generosity and dedication to community cultural interest—the cultural commonweal. Scholarly publication in the humanities, and even in poetry and other creative literary works, has been sustained in important measure by university presses. Private studio schools and academic centers of music, art, and drama have increasingly become the wellsprings of innovative creativity. They have nurtured imaginative work that found support solely from the returns of the commercial box office.

In the vast area of scientific advance in medicine as well as the delivery of health care, private foundations, universities, and great nonacademic clinical centers have fostered innovations in medicine, nursing, and hospital care. In the search for new and better ways to organize and finance health care, the names of Rockefeller, Sloan, Kaiser, and Johnson come to mind.

Perhaps the greatest and most pervasive contribution of the nonprofit sector in this great public cause of national health has been the development of insurance and prepayment through the establishment and evolution of Blue Cross and Blue Shield. I leave it to others, far more expert and experienced than I, to prescribe and forecast what the role of government, private fee-for-service, and nonprofit organization should be and will be in the fifty years ahead. Suffice it for me to assert the obvious—that the achievement and maintenance of the nation's health is a national purpose that will require a constant experimentation by all three sectors—the public, the market, and the nonprofit.

I have suggested that in addition to the values of localism, variety, and community purpose that the voluntary sector affords, there are some activities of crucial importance to the nation that inherently defy an exclusively public or an exclusively profit-oriented approach. Education, particularly at the level of advanced training and research, cannot be governed solely by tests of either political or marketplace popularity. The same is inherently true of the arts: If they are to be truly creative, they must be free to defy the inherited conventions or the distraction of profitable fads. And neither the market nor government can be the sole determinant of health care if the fiduciary obligation of the doctor and the relative helplessness of the patient are to be given adequate consideration. Neither the laws of supply and demand nor the laws of political accountability will be sufficient to govern these three areas. All of them require an active and significant role for a diverse and autonomous nonprofit sector.

However, for all three—education, the arts, and health care—it is now accepted that public financial assistance is also indispensable. This need is compounded by persistent inflation that outpaces private sources of support. As a recent supplicant for government funds for the arts and humanities, as well as for science and medicine, far be it from me to begrudge such public outlays simply because I find myself temporarily on the public payroll.

However, it is not inappropriate to assert as loudly and clearly as possible that public support of the voluntary sector must be in the spirit of investment in private initiative in the public interest. It is investment in the process by which free citizens and independent organizations seek to pursue truth, encourage creativity, and improve the human condition. It is not the procurement by contract of a given quantity of education, truth, art, or health. Government as investor must be willing to risk the variety of styles, approaches, and organizations that are the special strength of the voluntary sector. If, in order to avoid the chance of failure, government tries to direct the voluntary private initiative, let alone tries to prescribe how private groups shall go about their work, it will squeeze out the vitality of dispersed initiative that makes public investment worth the taxpayers' money in the first place.

It is precisely in order to encourage private initiative in the public interest, free from the heavy hand of centralized direction, that we take the biggest calculated risk of all—the tax deduction for charitable and educational purposes. It is not to indulge the whim of the taxpayer, but because we are convinced that the public interest will be better served by the pluralism, the commitment to community purposes, and the commitment of individual initiative, that we forego substantial revenue to encourage the private pursuit of the public interest.

So, I return to my starting point, the original American dream of a voluntary society.

This vision inspired the War of Independence. It guided the constitutional architects who sought to protect localism and diversity by constructing a federal system, reserving to the states those powers not vested in the central government. It has also been the glory of our reliance on private initiative in a free market as the best way to develop the enormous potential of our continent. With all its imperfections and inequities, this willingness to rely on a dispersion of political and economic power has made us the most truly voluntary society in the history of humanity.

In the fifty years ahead, the inevitable bigness of government and business, the inevitable impersonality of larger and more complex organizations in both the public and the private sector are perhaps the greatest challenge to our effort to make life as voluntary as possible for all citizens. In addition, as government becomes bigger and more pervasive, it badly needs to be tested and held to account by the standards of a private yardstick. Finally, there are areas crucial to the quality of any society—its education, its culture, and its health—that cannot be adequately nurtured if left solely to either the ballot box or the marketplace. As one British friend has put it, "Your country and mine have long known that the public interest is much too important to leave to the government."

UNFINISHED BUSINESS FOR THE
HEALTH CARE SYSTEM

Patricia Roberts Harris
Secretary, U.S. Department of Health
and Human Services

When Justin Ford Kimball conceived the idea of prepaid hospital insurance fifty years ago, the state of the nation's health was quite different from what it is today. The popular historian William Manchester said, in describing the conditions that existed at that time, "There were no sulfa drugs and no antibiotics. Meningitis killed 95 percent of its victims; pneumonia was often fatal. Even viral infections (called 'the grippe' then) were a serious business. Though hospitals were comparatively inexpensive, practically no one had hospital insurance, so most patients remained at home and seldom had the help of medication."

There have been revolutionary advances in medical research since that time, but success in the laboratory does not by itself improve the health of the population. Making improved health care available to people is equally important, and no group deserves more credit for accepting that challenge than Blue Cross and Blue Shield. Fifty years later, the general health of the American people has never been better. That conclusion is drawn from the report, "Health United States 1979," which was submitted to Congress by the Public Health Service in December 1979. We can all take pride in the progress it cites:

We are living longer—much longer—than we were just a few short decades ago. The average lifespan today is 73.2 years—nearly three years longer than it was a decade ago and twelve years longer than it was when Blue Cross was founded.

Our infant mortality rate is at its lowest point in history. Furthermore, we have reduced the mortality rate for children between ages one and fourteen by one-half in just the last generation.

Infectious diseases like polio, diphtheria, German measles, and whooping cough have either disappeared or been dramatically reduced. Smallpox—once one of the most vicious and dreaded diseases—has been eradicated.

Cardiovascular mortality rates have plummeted 22 percent in the last decade, and the incidence of stroke is down by 32 percent.

That essentially bright picture is clouded, however, by other evidence, which indicates that much remains to be done before we can say with confidence that our health care system is sound. Despite our progress, we have some unfinished business, primarily in four specific areas that must have special attention as we enter the 1980s: cost, coverage, disease prevention, and changing needs.

The cost of this nation's health care system is too high. Total expenditures for health have risen to more than $200 billion a year, almost 10 percent of the gross national product, and they continue to rise at a pace that far outstrips the inflation rate. Federal health costs alone will be well over $50 billion in 1980—nearly 12 percent of a total federal budget—that includes more than $30 billion for Medicare and an estimated $12 billion for Medicaid. We could live with the current price tag on health care if it resulted in quality care that would not be available for less. But that is not the case. We now know that we can lower costs and improve medical care, both at the same time.

The availability of care is also a major concern. Nearly 50 million of our fellow citizens, most of them poor, live in urban or rural settings that are medically underserved. More than 37 million Americans—again, most of them poor—have inadequate health insurance or no health insurance at all. More than 10 million children covered by Medicaid are entitled to health care only after they become sick. For them, preventive care and early screening for disease are too rare.

It is, in Charles Dickens' classic phrase, "The best of times and the worst of times." If you happen to be well-to-do, if you have purchased health insurance, and if you live in an area where quality care is available, your chances for a healthy life are better today than they have ever been before. For others the situation is not as hopeful. For black Americans between the ages of twenty-five and forty-four, for instance, the death rate is nearly two and a half times as great as it is for whites in the same age category. The infant mortality rate for blacks is twice as high as it is for whites. And a black male can anticipate a life eight years shorter than his white counterpart. Those conditions are not acceptable. A nation as rich and resourceful as ours can, and must, do better.

The third area that requires our serious attention is the allocation of the federal health dollar. Earlier, I cited statistics that highlighted the success we have had in treating a number of serious diseases. We have achieved that success largely because we have committed tremendous resources to the effort—a commitment, I might add, that is virtually unique in the world. It is now time to ask, however, if we should continue the level of funding allocated in recent years for disease treatment, or whether we should redirect some of that money to the area of disease prevention.

The biggest killer today is cardiovascular disease, and we have learned that such factors as smoking and nutrition can have a striking effect on its incidence. Smoking and environmental factors are also important in the case of cancer, the second most deadly menace. We might be able to lower the incidence of even this disease by concentrating on these areas.

Fourth, and finally, demographers tell us that our population is changing. As the average lifespan grows longer, and as the birth rate holds at a relatively low rate, several things are happening. The proportion of older people in our population is increasing, and when the post–World War II baby boom reaches retirement age, the absolute number of older people will also enlarge dramatically. But the most significant improvement in the area of longevity has been among those who have already reached their fifties and sixties. This means we will see an ever greater number of our fellow citizens living into their eighth and ninth decades. People at that age often have very special needs and concerns, and we must prepare now for increases in that population.

These four concerns are among the most prominent challenges we face today, and they dictate much of the agenda for the coming decade. First, we must find some way to slow the inflation rate in health costs. That is why the Carter administration has proposed an effective hospital cost containment bill and why we will continue to fight hard for the passage of legislation that accomplishes these ends. Strong hospital cost containment legislation is critically important in the battle against inflation, and it is an important goal for those of us concerned about the availability of health care to all our citizens. It must be achieved, and I am confident that it will be.

We will also seek other remedies, such as strengthening health maintenance organizations, in order to develop a health care system that is more efficient, less costly, and provides wider choice for the patient.

Expanding the health care system to include all our citizens is an equally difficult task, but we have begun that effort as well. We in the Carter administration have worked to make yearly periodic screening, diagnosis, and treatment programs for Medicaid children more effective. We have doubled the number of federally funded community health centers in just two years. We have more than doubled the National Health Service Corps. We have proposed the Child Health Assurance Program to expand Medicaid coverage to an additional 2 million poor children and 100,000 pregnant women, and we have built in incentives to encourage increased preventive and primary care for these patients. Finally, we have proposed a workable national health plan that would provide all Americans, through employment-based or public plans, with protection against catastrophic medical expenses—protection that 83 million of our citizens lack today.

The national health plan would provide fully subsidized and comprehensive coverage to nearly 16 million low-income people not now eligible for Medicaid by establishing a minimum income level below which all persons would be covered. The national health plan also would improve the health care system by increasing competition and containing costs.

These are, in President Carter's words, times of "hard choices and scarce resources," but they are not times to stand still. The Carter national health plan can be enacted, and it can serve as the foundation for a more equitable health system in this country, but it will need support.

The strategy in the third area, disease prevention, is found in the recent surgeon general's report. We can, and we will, reallocate some of our resources in order to strengthen emphasis on the prevention of disease. We have established goals for the coming decade that will require greater emphasis on preventive health services, health education, and environmental controls.

As we discover new trends, we have a responsibility to prepare the health system to meet the needs of an older population. This will require careful study in a number of areas. The Department of Health and Human Services, for instance, has already initiated programs to help us determine how long-term care services, both institutional and home-based, can be improved in preparation for the greater role they will play in the years ahead.

That leads to a final point, one that is essential to the success of all our efforts. Government cannot alone create a strong health care system. The private sector alone cannot extend that system to include all Americans, especially the most vulnerable in our society. It will take the combined efforts of government and private organizations, most notably the Blue Cross and Blue Shield organization, if Americans are to be healthier and free from fear of health care costs in the years to come. We need to renew and enhance the spirit of partnership that has developed throughout the last half-century. We will have differences of opinion, and that is to be expected, but we must be ready to work out those differences, placing first the greater goal of service to the public.

It has become a clich´e to say something is at a crossroads—education, the economy, and every aspect of foreign policy seem to be found there perpetually. Still, the health care system *has* reached a crossroads. Anyone who reads the newspapers and follows the nightly news knows we have many options, but I can assure you that the status quo is not among them. The health system will change—must change—and I hope we can work together to change it. More than thirty years ago, President Harry Truman saw the issue: "Millions of our citizens," he said, "do not now have a full measure of opportunity to achieve and to enjoy good health. Millions do not now have protection or security against the economic effects of sickness."

Despite our progress in recent years, much of what President Truman said remains true today. As we approach the beginning of a new decade, certainly the time has now arrived for action. Let us meet that challenge together, renewing our partnership in service to the American people.

Reference

Manchester, W. 1974. *The Glory and the Dream: A Narrative History of America, 1932–1972.* Boston: Little, Brown & Co.

A STEP-BY-STEP APPROACH TO HEALTH

Stuart E. Eizenstat
Assistant to the President for
Domestic Affairs and Policy

In order to understand and make judgments about the federal administration proposal and other proposals in the health-financing area, I believe it is imperative to begin with a review of the problems that we feel health care-financing proposals must address. In putting together the administration's national health plan, we identified three sets of problems within our current health care and health-financing systems.

The first set of problems is a lack of adequate insurance coverage under our present public and private systems. The most recent figures available to us indicate that some 22 million Americans have no health insurance protection at all. An additional 20 million have grossly inadequate health insurance coverage by almost anybody's standards. These people, by and large, have very inadequate individual policies, with many exclusions, preexisting condition limitations, and very low payout ratios. In addition to these roughly 42 million Americans with either no coverage or grossly inadequate coverage, an additional 41 million have inadequate protection against the costs of major catastrophic illnesses.

The second set of problems we identified was the issue of rapidly rising health care costs. This problem has received a great deal of attention over recent years. I will not repeat the entire litany of numbers; suffice it to say that total health care costs in 1979 are equivalent to 9.1 percent of the gross national product, or $206 billion, and we predict a rise to 10.2 percent of the GNP, or $368 billion, by 1984—unless corrective actions are taken. Health care costs currently account for 12.7 percent of the federal budget, or some $62 billion, and are projected to rise steeply to 14.5 percent of the budget, or $110 billion, in 1984, without adequate legislative changes. These figures hold a very clear message—namely, that developing a national health-financing plan without appropriate cost containment measures would be a most irresponsible endeavor, and that any health plan must be based on adequate provisions to contain increases in health care costs.

While many forces have conspired to create these unacceptable increases in health care costs, let me focus on those caused by the current health-financing system—forces that health insurers as an industry have the greatest leverage to change. The rise in costs stems primarily from inefficiencies in the current system, resulting from the absence of traditional competitive market forces:

- More than 90 percent of all hospital bills are paid by third parties, including private insurance companies, Blue Cross, and the federal government. Neither the consumer (the patient) nor the provider (the doctor and the hospital industry) directly feel the pinch of rising costs.
- These third parties, in the private sector and in the federal government, in part, customarily pay for services to beneficiaries on a cost-plus basis for hospital care and on the basis of physician-determined charges for medical services.
- Customary interactions between buyers and sellers do not take place in the health care market. Most decisions are made by the provider, not the consumer. Physicians control more than 70 percent of health care decisions.

The increase in health care costs resulting from these forces was the principal reason for this administration's hospital cost containment proposal. The unique anticompetitive nature of this industry has prompted this regulatory approach by an administration that has clearly established itself as pro-deregulation in many other industries, including trucking and airlines.

I do not mean to imply that we believe the regulatory approach is the only long-term solution to the problem. This administration actively supports and encourages innovative financing, reimbursement, and delivery systems—such as health maintenance organizations (HMOs) and individual practice associations (IPAs)—to change these market forces that create inefficiency and result in the inflation we are now experiencing.

The burden of reform cannot, and should not, rest solely with the federal government, however. There is plenty of room for improving the current private reimbursement system by changing the inflationary and perverse incentive it creates, including current incentives for doctors to provide specialty care as opposed to less costly primary care, incentives to provide hospital care in lieu of less costly outpatient care, and the lack of incentives to practice in those areas where health care is most desperately needed. These incentives have created the third set of problems that we identified—insufficient emphasis on prevention, primary care, and outpatient services; and the fact that some 50 million Americans live in medically underserved areas.

These, then, were the problems we sought to deal with as we put together our national health plan. Since the outset of his campaign for the presidency five years ago, President Carter has consistently stated his belief that we should ultimately have in this country a system that protects all citizens against the costs of a comprehensive range of health care services. In each of his statements on this issue he has also stressed his firm belief that such coverage must be very carefully phased in if we are to avoid adverse effects on the federal budget and the economy in general, and the kind of administrative nightmares that resulted from the attempt to implement rapidly such programs as Medicaid in the mid-1960s.

Our task, then, was to develop a step-by-step approach that would begin to deal with the most serious of the problems I have described, and at the same time not produce a negative impact on the federal budget and the economy as a whole. We believe that the plan that we have developed meets those tests and represents a realistic and responsible starting point for serious congressional debate.

The plan has three major components. The first of these is the employer mandate component, under which we would mandate that all employers provide health insurance coverage to their employees. There are three significant points to make about that mandated coverage.

1. All policies would have to meet a series of conditions that would line up the "fine print" in health insurance policies.

For example, we would mandate coverage of school-attending dependents up to age twenty-two or twenty-six, coverage for ninety days after unemployment, and so on. These provisions are most important, for they would result in closing some of the most significant gaps in coverage that exist today.

2. Under the employer mandate, all policies would have to cover a comprehensive range of benefits—although in the first-phase plan, policies could have a deductible of up to $2,500. In other words, those employers who offer no coverage today would be mandated under our plan to offer *at a minimum* adequate major-medical coverage. This is perhaps the outstanding feature of our first-phase plan that differentiates it from other universal, comprehensive proposals. It represents the most specific example of where we attempted to balance carefully the benefit protection that we felt was necessary against the demands that added benefits could place upon the economy. For example, our estimates showed that if we were to mandate that those employers who currently offered no coverage move immediately to offering a fully comprehensive package without deductibles or coinsurance, the premium for such coverage in 1980 could be over $2,000 per family. Our estimates showed that that kind of burden could result in a loss of up to one million jobs and an increase in the inflation rate of 1-1/2 percent. By limiting the mandate to major-medical coverage in our plan, we were able to drop that premium to the range of $500 per year per family and therefore significantly reduce the impact on the economy.

3. We included a special provision under which all plans would cover care for infants up to the age of one and pregnant women without the application of a deductible. These provisions were included so that we could begin at the outset to build the soundest possible base of financing for that group in the population for whom early and preventive services are of the utmost importance.

As a result of the employer mandate, the dollar volume of sales by private health insurance companies would increase by 12 percent, from $59 to $66 billion. In addition, private insurers would administer claims payments on behalf of the plan, handling $55 billion in benefit payments.

The second major component of the plan is the establishment of a new public program, which we have labeled "Healthcare." I would make two points about Healthcare. First, this program would combine the existent Medicare and Medicaid programs into one program for the aged, the poor, the disabled, and other citizens who have difficulty obtaining coverage in the private market. The plan would be federally administered, using private insurers as carriers and intermediaries on a competitive bid basis. Second, under this component of our bill, we would substantially expand coverage for the low-income population. There are major gaps in coverage of the low-income population under the current Medicaid program. For example, it is restricted to welfare families, so that intact "working poor" families, singles, and childless couples are not eligible for coverage at all. Under our plan, we would cover an additional 14 million low-income citizens and establish a floor of protection so that all of the very poorest of our citizens would be fully covered at the outset of our program.

The third major component of our proposal is a series of cost control and system reform provisions. Two of the cost control provisions are most worthy of note. First, our proposal incorporates the hospital reimbursement provisions encompassed in our hospital cost containment legislation. Responsible hospital cost containment legislation has thus far not been passed by the Congress. We hope that the Congress will see the error of its way over the next year. In any event, as critical as is the current need for such legislation, it would be compounded with additional health insurance coverage. We are confident that almost every member of the Congress could grasp the need for responsible hospital reimbursement mechanisms in the context of health insurance legislation that would add billions of dollars to public and private expenditures for health care services.

The second major cost control provision deals with physician reimbursement. Here again, we felt strongly that it would be irresponsible to develop a national health proposal that would pay physicians their billed charges on an open-ended, blank-check basis. In examining the alternatives, we felt that a fee schedule based on average Medicare reimbursements in each area of the country would represent the most responsible approach to physician reimbursement under the Healthcare program. I should point out that in developing that fee schedule we would raise the Medicaid reimbursement (which in many states has been too low) up to the Medicare level, thereby substantially increasing payments to physicians under the public programs—and providing an additional incentive for doctors to treat Medicaid patients.

We decided to limit the mandatory application of the fee schedule to the Healthcare, or public, program, rather than extending it to the private, or employer-mandate, part of the program, but we would send those fee schedules to all insurers and make them available to the public in each area of the country. Our belief is that this benchmark, set by the public plan, will allow consumers to make more-informed decisions in choosing their providers and will give insurers leverage to develop alternative, innovative, and noninflationary mechanisms for reimbursing physicians.

With respect to system reform, there are again two major sets of provisions. The first is aimed at increasing competition within the Healthcare system. Under these provisions, we would improve reimbursement for HMOs under the public program, mandate that employers offer multiple choices of plans, and require that employers make equal contributions to the plans so that the consumer can feel the impact of cost-effective choices. In the area of prevention, the most important provision is the universal coverage, with comprehensive benefits, for children and pregnant women.

In summary then, the administration's plan consists of three major components: employer-mandate major-medical coverage, the establishment of Healthcare to improve substantially coverage of the low-income population, and a series of cost control and system reform provisions. We believe firmly that this plan represents a realistic, responsible starting point for congressional deliberation. We believe it is a responsible middle ground between proposals—such as catastrophic-only coverage—too narrow to deal effectively with the problems I have outlined and proposals so broad as to be harmful to the economy, difficult to administer, and, as has been shown for thirty years, impossible to pass.

The first type, the catastrophic proposals, deals only with the high costs of major illness. Although we recognize the political appeal and lower cost of this type of proposal and affirm catastrophic coverage as a real need, we feel that such proposals pose three significant dangers. First, catastrophic coverage alone would lead to an escalation of unnecessary expenditure for high-cost, high-technology care, unless it were to be combined with adequate reimbursement, utilization, and technology controls.

Second, passage of only a catastrophic bill would not be equitable. Millions of poor and elderly citizens would be driven to financial despair before even qualifying for coverage. Third, a catastrophic-only bill will not establish a framework for realizing our ultimate goal—universal, comprehensive health protection, including preventive and primary-care services, for *all* Americans.

The other major type of proposal, which promises very broad public coverage within a very short period of time, poses equally severe problems. Such a proposal is completely antagonistic to the fundamental concerns of the public and their representatives in Congress. Given the level of anxiety about inflation, a major and sudden increase in federal spending will not have popular support. It would also steal resources from other domestic areas—employment and training, education, mass transit, and energy. Considering the degree of concern about federal government overregulation, a proposal for a new, intrusive, and dominating role for the federal government would also not have much popular support. Our proposal avoids these problems by building constructively on current public and private insurance programs and by being carefully phased in to minimize the burden on the economy.

We were very pleased to see that the Senate Finance Committee began markup sessions on health insurance legislation in late 1979. I applaud the leadership of Chairman Russell Long, and the actions of the committee in moving rapidly on this issue are encouraging. So far, the committee has dealt primarily with decisions about coverage of the employed population. Although we have some reservations about various provisions they have tentatively approved, the employer-mandate portion of the finance committee plan is reasonably similar to the administration's plan. I want to reaffirm the commitment of this administration to a national health plan that provides assistance to all Americans and that deals responsibly with the need for cost containment. *A catastrophic-coverage-only plan will not be acceptable, nor will a plan that does not include strong cost controls and incentives for efficient health care delivery.* I believe that many members of the finance committee support this position.

INDEX

About the Contributors

WILLIAM G. ANLYAN, M.D., is vice president for health affairs at Duke University, where he is also professor of surgery. He is a former chairman of the Association of American Medical Colleges.

KINGMAN BREWSTER, JR., U.S. ambassador to the United Kingdom, was formerly president of Yale University.

EDWARD J. CONNORS is president of the Sisters of Mercy Health Corporation at Farmington Hills, Michigan.

JOHN A. D. COOPER, M.D., is president of the Association of American Medical Colleges. He is also professor of health policy at Duke University and consultant to the National Institutes of Health.

RICHARD H. EGDAHL, M.D., is director of the Health Policy Institute at Boston University, where he has also been professor and chairman of the department of surgery.

STUART E. EIZENSTAT is on the White House staff as assistant to the president for domestic affairs and policy. He was a policy adviser to Mr. Carter during the 1976 presidential campaign and formerly practiced law in Atlanta.

RASHI FEIN, Ph.D., is professor of health economics at Harvard Medical School and is the author of books on medical economics, medical education, and national health policy.

DONALD S. FREDRICKSON, M.D., is director of the National Institutes of Health and a member of the faculties in preventive medicine at both the George Washington University and Georgetown University schools of medicine.

LAWRENCE W. GREEN, Dr. P.H., is director of the Office of Health Information, Health Promotion, Physical Fitness and Sports in the U.S. Department of Health and Human Services. He was formerly professor in, and head of, the division of health education at the Johns Hopkins school of hygiene and public health.

DAVID A. HAMBURG, M.D., is president of the Institute of Medicine, National Academy of Sciences. He was formerly professor in, and head of, the department of psychiatry at Stanford University Medical School.

PATRICIA R. HARRIS is secretary of the U.S. Department of Health and Human Services. She was previously secretary of the Department of Housing and Urban Development.

WALTER J. McNERNEY is president of the Blue Cross and Blue Shield Associations. He was formerly professor in, and director of, the Bureau of Health Administration at the University of Michigan.

EDMUND D. PELLEGRINO, M.D., is president of the Catholic University of America in Washington, D.C. He was formerly president of the Yale-New Haven Medical Center and professor of medicine at Yale University school of medicine.

JULIUS B. RICHMOND, M.D., is assistant secretary of the U.S. Department of Health and Human Services and surgeon general of the Public Health Service. He was formerly professor and chairman of the department of preventive and social medicine at Harvard Medical School.

IRVING J. SELIKOFF, M.D., is professor of medicine, professor and chairman of the division of environmental medicine, and director of the environmental sciences laboratory at the Mount Sinai school of medicine, New York City.

MARVIN J. SHAPIRO, M.D., former chairman of Blue Shield of California, is a member of the Joint Executive Committee of the Blue Cross and Blue Shield Associations. He is a practicing radiologist in Encino, California.

VICTOR W. SIDEL, M.D., is professor of community health and chairman of the department of social medicine at Albert Einstein college of medicine, New York City. He is also professor of health, medicine, and society at City University.

NATHAN J. STARK is undersecretary of the U.S. Department of Health and Human Services. He was formerly vice chancellor of the schools of the health professions at the University of Pittsburgh and president of the University Medical Center.

MALCOLM C. TODD, M.D., practices surgery in Long Beach, California, and is a former president of the American Medical Association. He is clinical professor of surgery at the University of California at Irvine and is a trustee of the Long Beach Memorial Hospital Medical Center.